"Recent science about our emotions has shown t
This wonderful book is full of great examples, fur
activities. It's friendly, inviting, and fun—and very effective. A gem!"

—**Rick Hanson, PhD,** author of *Hardwiring Happiness*

"The Big Book of Big Feelings is a fun and creative approach to help kids actively identify emotions in themselves and others, boosting their emotional intelligence."

—**Tina Payne Bryson, PhD,** *New York Times* bestselling coauthor of *The Whole-Brain Child* and *The Way of Play*

"Rachael has created reading and writing activities that are kid friendly. This resource would be helpful for social-emotional learning (SEL) with a parent or teacher. The graphics and real-world examples make it easy to engage a child."

—**Anna Jenkins,** principal at Alexander Adaire School in Philadelphia, PA

"As an integrative medicine physician, I understand how important healthy emotions are to a healthy person—and the earlier the start, the stronger the foundation for a healthy life. Rachael Katz's *The Big Book of Big Feelings* offers a brilliantly playful resource that invites children to explore their inner worlds with curiosity, safety, and empowerment. Complete with activity pages and stepwise guidance, this workbook can enhance any home or school."

—**Cynthia Li, MD,** doctor, and best-selling author of *Brave New Medicine*

"Fun is sticky. I only wish that in all my years, I had such a fun, engaging, interactive tool to help my young students navigate their feelings! Rachael has given us a gift. Kids will love their new friend Peep, his relatable examples, Rachael's own funny illustrations, and enticing prompts and carrots—all of which will keep them interested and probing and learning."

—**Sharon Leong,** teacher at Yu Ming Charter School, an award-winning Chinese immersion school in Oakland, CA

With *The Big Book of Big Feelings*, Rachael Katz brings us the endearing 'Peep,' who will have readers and pre-readers identifying, exploring, and understanding their emotions. From the get-go, Peep appeals with his sense of humor and humility, especially as he invites young ones to take the driver's seat. Expect meaningful engagement and a request for more Peep!"

—**Gail Silver, E-RYT, RCYT, JD,** founder of Yoga Child Inc., mindfulness educator, and award-winning author of *Anh's Anger* and other books for children

THE
BIG BOOK
OF
BIG
FEELINGS

AN EMOTIONAL INTELLIGENCE ACTIVITY BOOK FOR KIDS

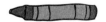

RACHAEL KATZ, MEd

Instant Help Books
An Imprint of New Harbinger Publications, Inc.

Publisher's Note

INSTANT HELP, the Clock Logo, and NEW HARBINGER are trademarks of New Harbinger Publications, Inc.

Distributed in Canada by Raincoast Books

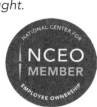

Copyright © 2025 by Rachael Katz
Instant Help Books
An imprint of New Harbinger Publications, Inc.
5720 Shattuck Avenue
Oakland, CA 94609
www.newharbinger.com

Cover design by Sara Christian. Cover illustrations by Rachael Katz.

Interior book design by Rachael Katz

Acquired by Ryan Buresh

Edited by Vicraj Gill

Printed in the United States of America

27   26   25

10   9   8   7   6   5   4   3   2   1

First Printing

To Jacob and Nina,
for being my constant inspiration
and greatest teachers.

And to all the amazing children I've had
the privilege to work with over the years—
thank you for sharing your feelings and
reminding me how important it is to listen.

LETTER TO READER

Hi there!

When you flip the page, you'll meet Peep, a little bird who really needs your help! To give Peep a hand, you'll get to read, write, and draw in this book. Look out for this symbol 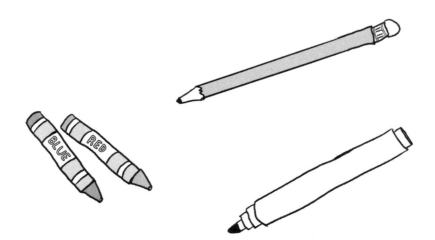 — it'll tell you what to do next!

So, grab your favorite markers, pens, pencils, or crayons, and get ready to dive in. Oh, and don't forget—there's a letter for adults at the back of the book. Make sure to remind them to read it!

Have fun!

TABLE OF CONTENTS

This book is so much fun!

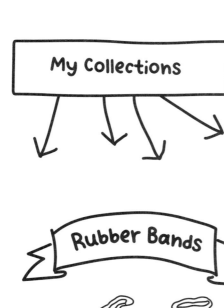

My Collections

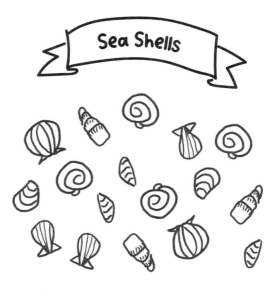

Sea Shells

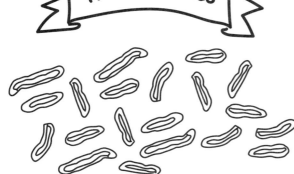

Rubber Bands

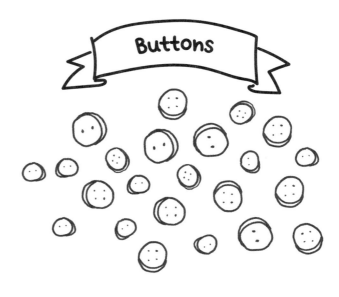

Buttons

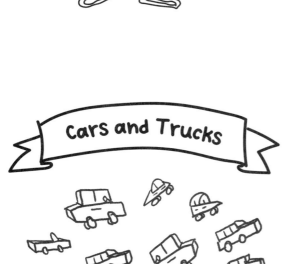

Cars and Trucks

Hello! I am Peep WGC—the World's Greatest Collector.

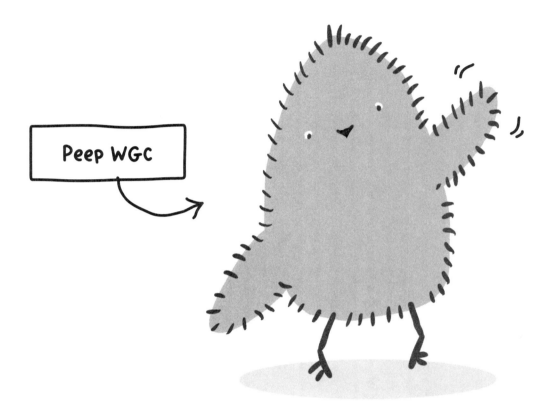

Peep WGC

My full name is William R. Peeples but everyone calls me Peep.

WGC stands for
World's Greatest Collector

(This is a name I made up. I got the idea from my teacher. He has letters after his name: Dr. Flippers, PhD.)

Right now, I'm working on a new collection. It'll be the greatest collection ever!

I collect things, big and small!

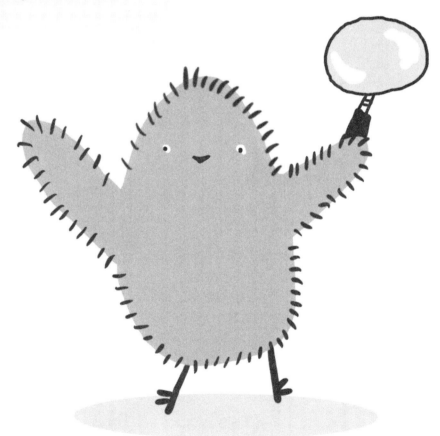

I got the idea last night at dinner when my Gran said,
"Peep, you sure are full of feelings!"

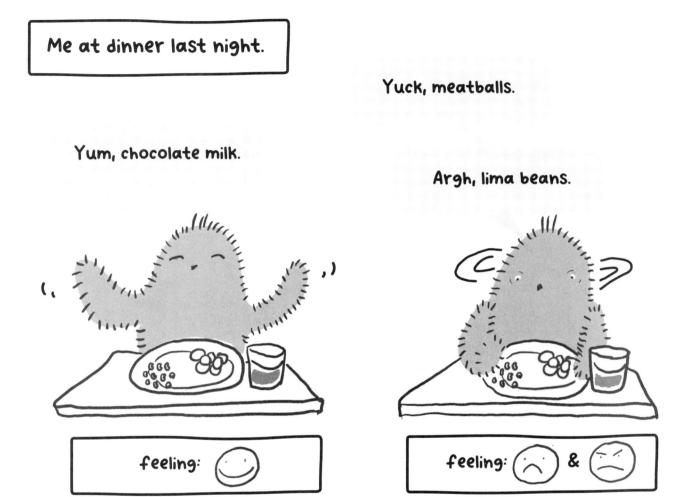

Me at dinner last night.

Yuck, meatballs.

Yum, chocolate milk.

Argh, lima beans.

feeling: 🙂

feeling: ☹ & 😠

If you're full of something, then you have a lot of it. And if you have a lot of something, you have a collection.

Gran said I was "full of feelings," so I have a new collection!

This collection is different. Most collections are made up of things—stuff you can touch, look at, smell, taste, and move. But this collection is invisible. There's nothing to see.

I made even more discoveries. Here they are:

(1.) Every feeling has a name, like "sad," "happy," or "angry."

(2.) Feelings make our bodies feel a certain way, like TIGHT, TINGLY, or JUMPY.

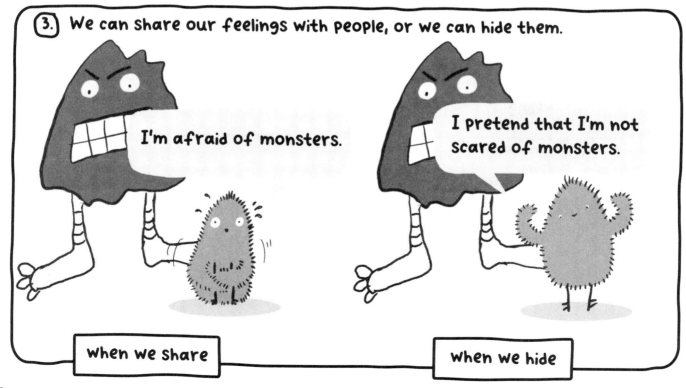

(3.) We can share our feelings with people, or we can hide them.

I'm afraid of monsters.

I pretend that I'm not scared of monsters.

when we share

when we hide

4.) Feelings can change quickly.

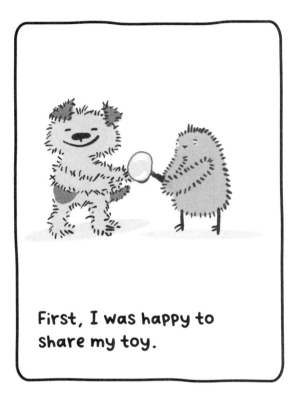

First, I was happy to share my toy.

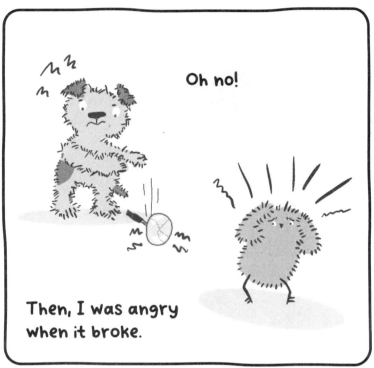

Oh no!

Then, I was angry when it broke.

5.) There are no right or wrong feelings.

6.) Feelings can be strong or weak.

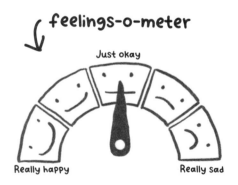

feelings-o-meter

Just okay

Really happy   Really sad

7.) We can have more than one feeling at the same time.

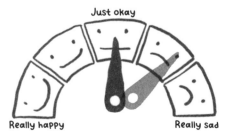

Just okay

Really happy   Really sad

I can only think of four feelings for the collection! How can I be the World's Greatest Collector of feelings with just four feeling words? My collection is too small!

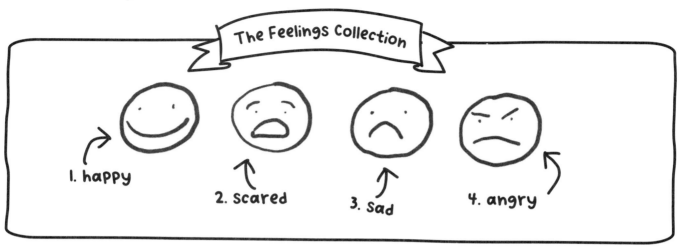

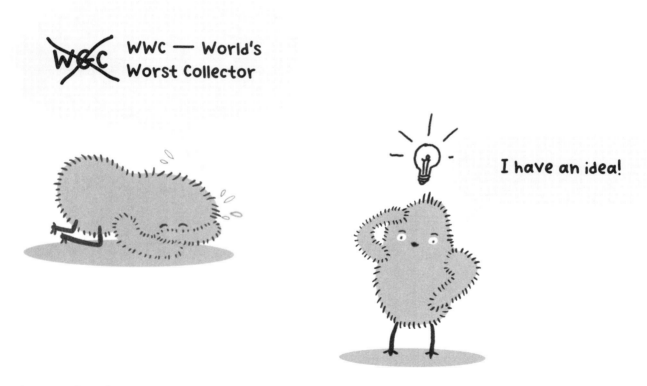

I need a friend and helper! Maybe you could help me? If you do, we could share the collection. We can be a team.

Here's how you can help. I'll tell you what happened to me last week, then you can name my feeling. We will be the greatest team ever.

And you know what? I really like you. So I'll let you be the World's Greatest Collector of feelings. I'll be the Second Best Collector of feelings. What do you think?

Write your name on the line. Decorate the award.

WORLD'S GREATEST COLLECTOR OF FEELINGS

#1

ARE YOU READY?

LET'S GET STARTED!

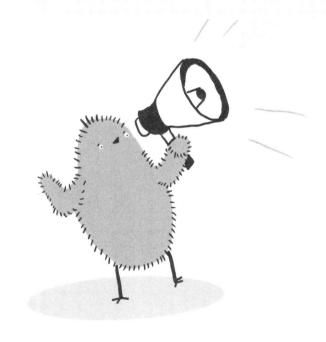

FIELD TRIP FIASCO

FEELING #5

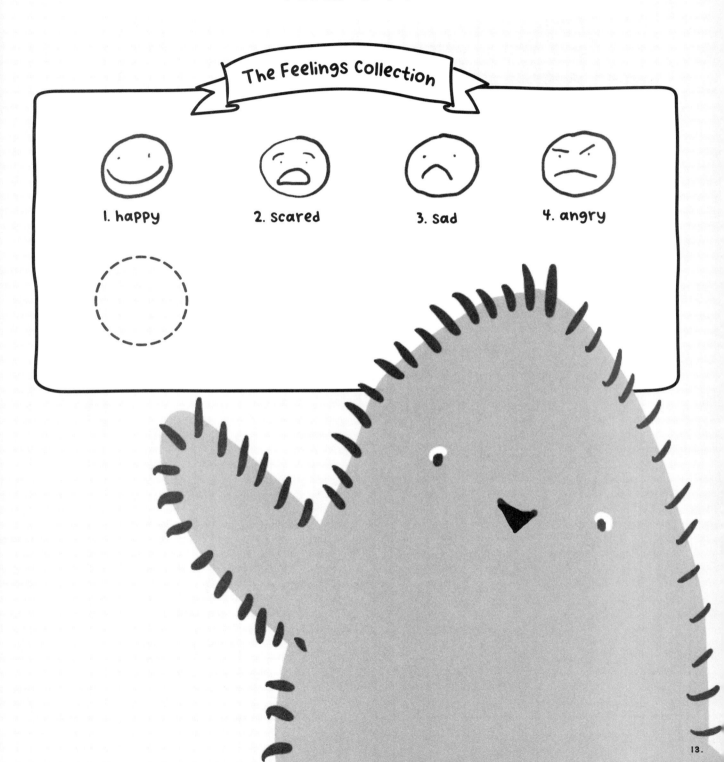

The Feelings Collection

1. happy
2. scared
3. sad
4. angry

On Monday, my class took a field trip to the science museum to look at bugs. I looked for mole crickets, my all-time favorite bug.*

There were no mole crickets. But there were lots of bugs eating food. Watching the bugs eat made me so hungry that my stomach started growling!

*

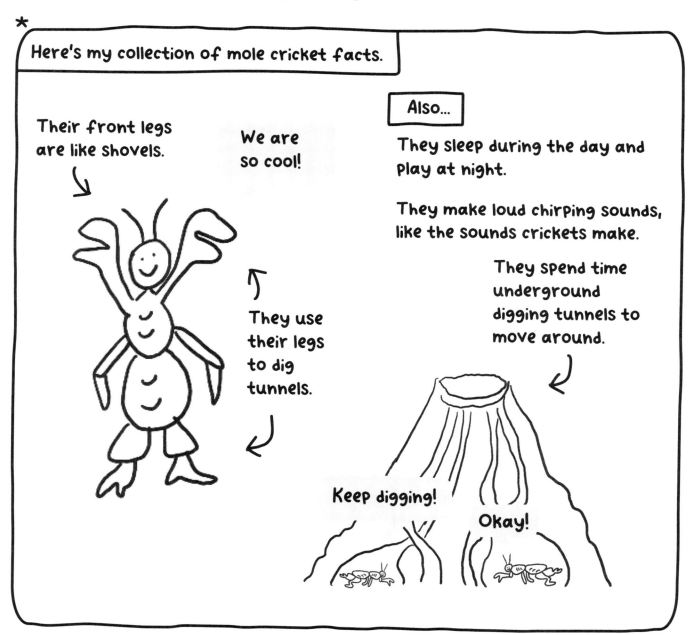

Here's my collection of mole cricket facts.

Their front legs are like shovels.

We are so cool!

They use their legs to dig tunnels.

Also...

They sleep during the day and play at night.

They make loud chirping sounds, like the sounds crickets make.

They spend time underground digging tunnels to move around.

Keep digging!

Okay!

By lunchtime, I was starving. I ate my food fast. When I opened my mouth to drink my juice, I burped loud!

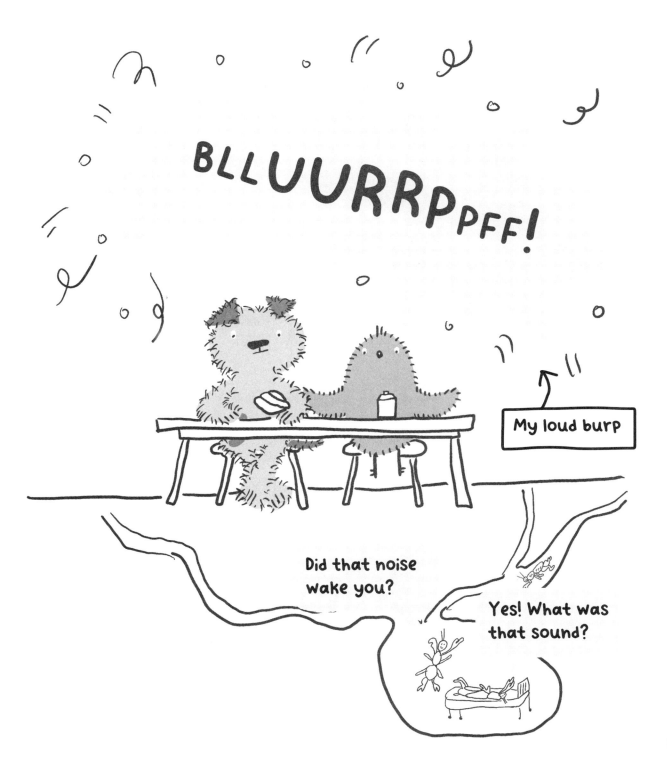

My class was shocked. Everyone stared at me. I wanted to dig a tunnel underground and hide with the mole crickets.

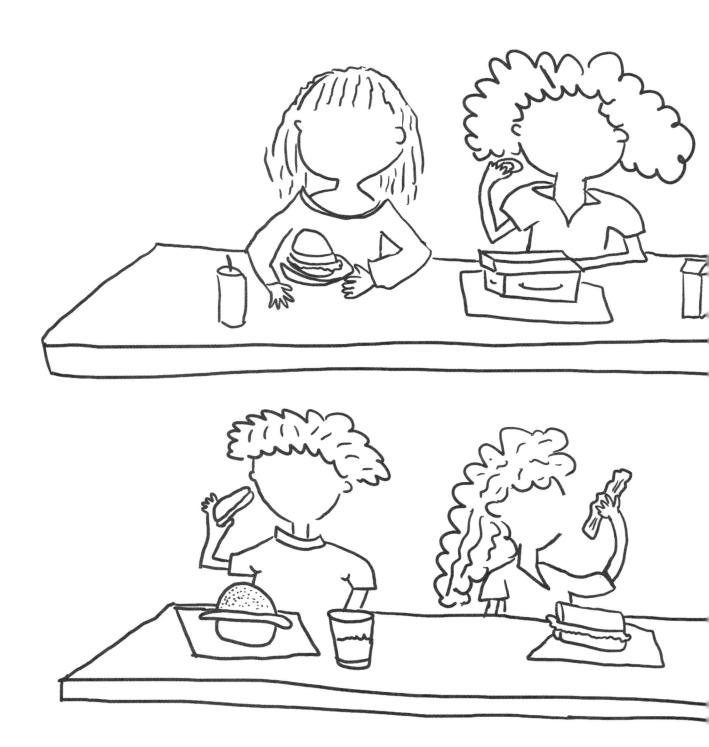

Do you know what it's like to be shocked?
Draw shocked faces.

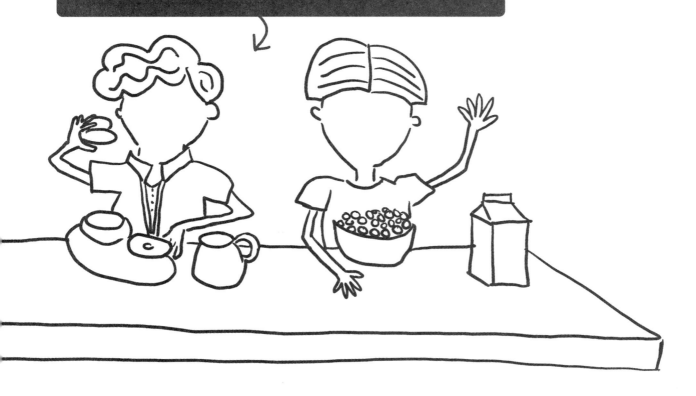

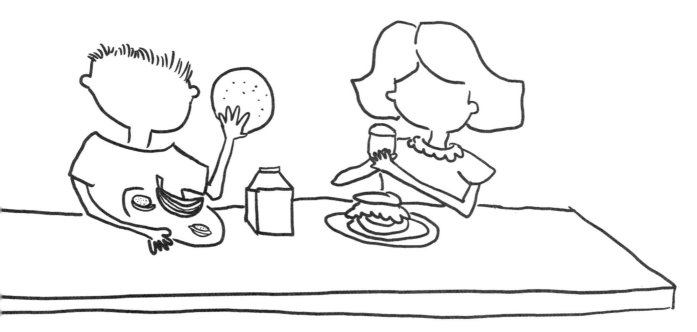

I was feeling....

_____

↗

Write the feeling on the line.

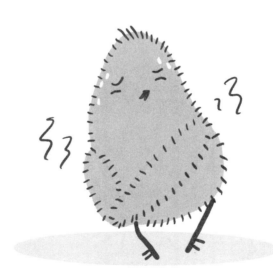

ANSWER: Embarrassed
Or other feelings—like ashamed

Good work, we named
the feeling!

Have you ever felt
embarrassed?

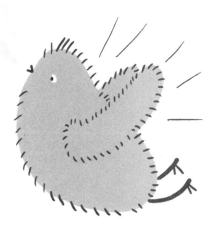

Write about or draw a time you felt embarrassed.

Draw the kids' embarrassed faces and their hair.

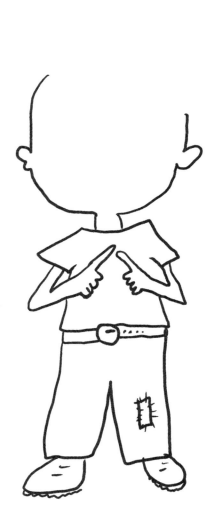

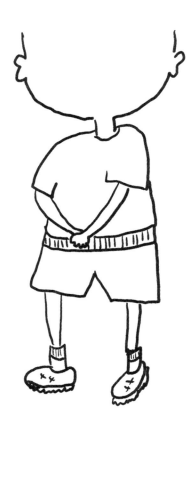

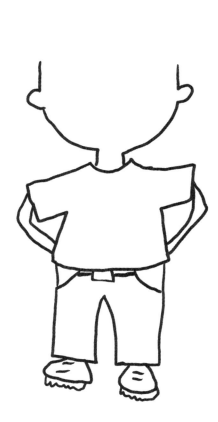

Circle the things that might make you feel embarrassed.

Auntie kissing you in front of your friends

Tripping and falling on the playground

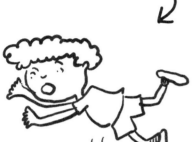

Your pants suddenly falling down

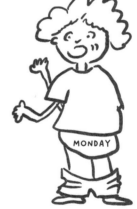

Having jam on your face all day

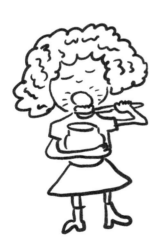

Farting out loud

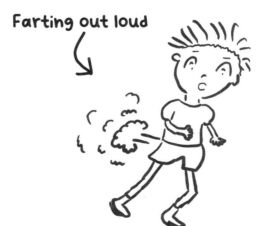

Peep's embarrassed and he wants to hide.
Follow the maze to help Peep hide.

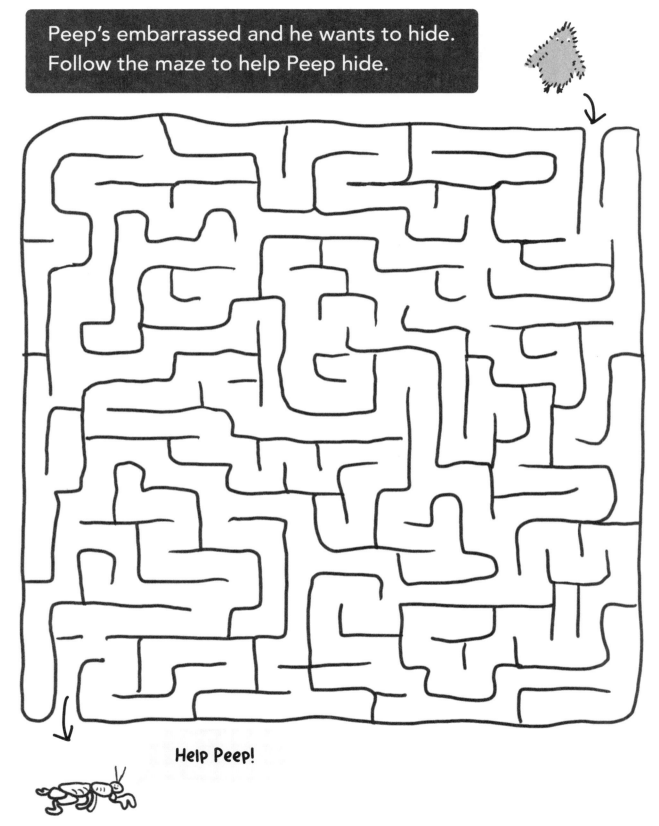

Help Peep!

Make up an embarrassing sound for each bubble.
Use the letters: T A R F B U P.

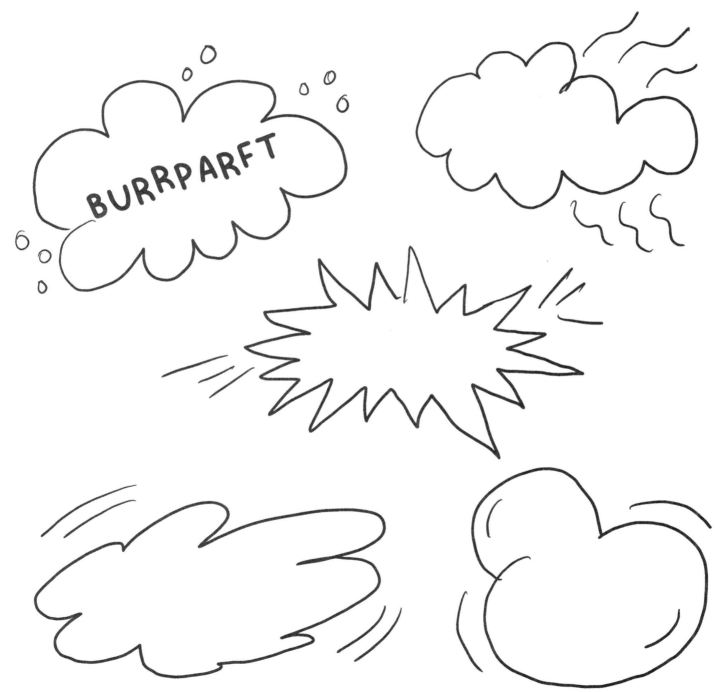

YOU'RE GREAT AT
NAMING FEELINGS!

YOU'RE ALSO GREAT AT
UNDERSTANDING WHAT THEY ARE!

ARE YOU READY TO
NAME THE NEXT ONE?

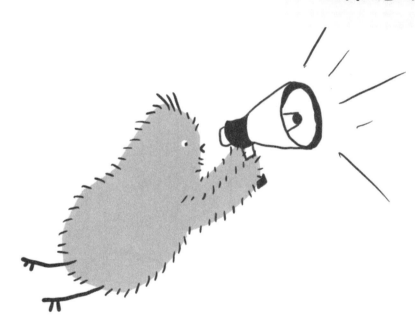

TREATS FOR CHAMPIONS
FEELING #6

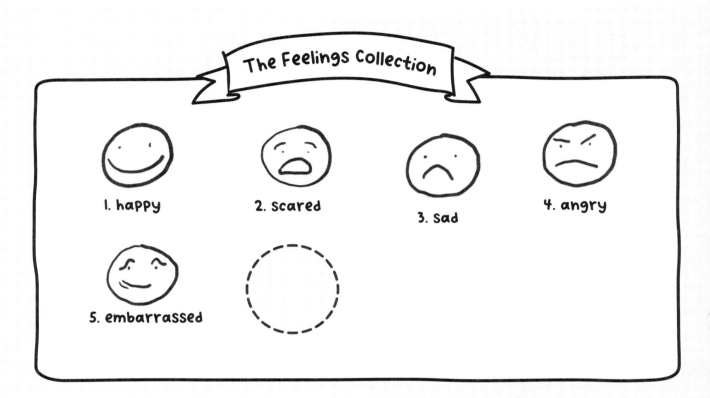

The Feelings Collection

1. happy
2. scared
3. Sad
4. angry
5. embarrassed

On Tuesday, I went to my swim lesson. Swimming didn't start out great. But Gran said I'd get a treat if I learned to swim.

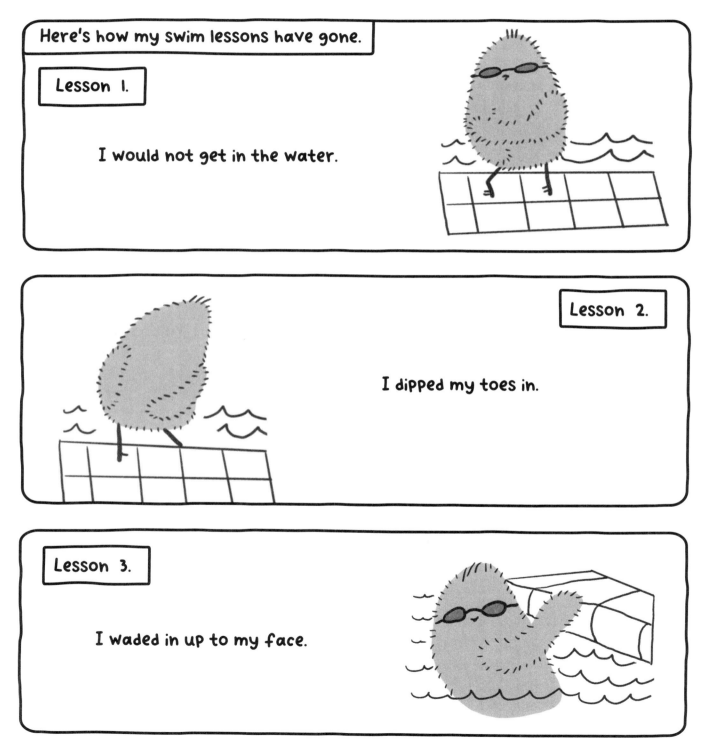

Here's how my swim lessons have gone.

Lesson 1.

I would not get in the water.

Lesson 2.

I dipped my toes in.

Lesson 3.

I waded in up to my face.

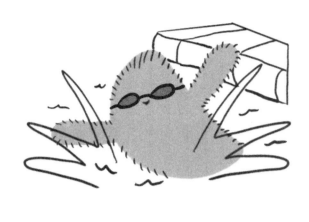

I dunked my face in the water for three seconds.

Lesson 5.

I did the chickie paddle. It's like the doggie paddle.

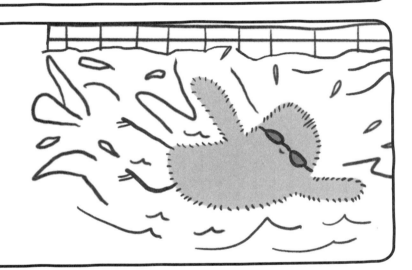

Lesson 6.

I swam across the pool on my own.

At the end of the lesson, Gran said I was a swim champ. Then she told me that swim champs get ice cream. I love ice cream!

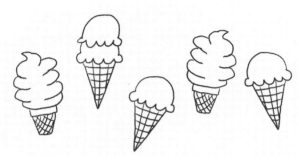

Which flavor?
I like so many!

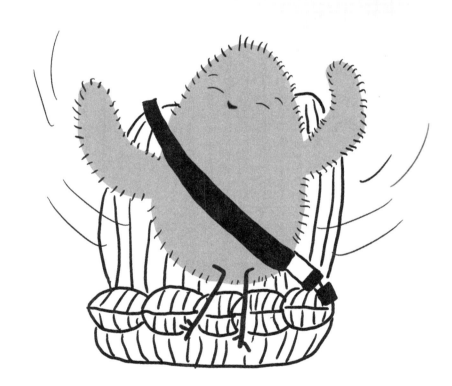

I bounced in the car on the way to the ice cream store. I couldn't stop bouncing.

Make Peep's favorite flavors. Add bugs and worms to the ice cream.

cookies and worms

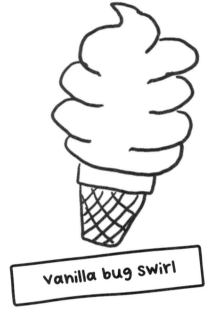

vanilla bug swirl

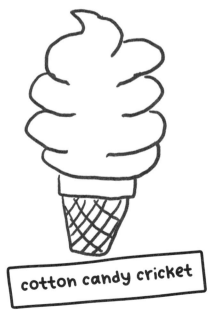

cotton candy cricket

mint chocolate ants

I was feeling….

_____

Write the feeling on the line.

Great job, we added another
feeling to the collection!

I think I had more than one
feeling at the same time.

Can you help me to name the other
feelings? You can write them
anywhere you want on this page.

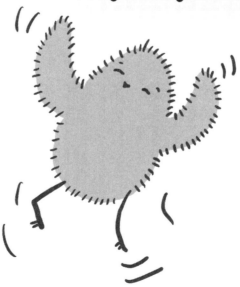

or other feelings—like thrilled or proud
ANSWER: Excited

Draw something that you would be really excited to find inside these gift boxes.

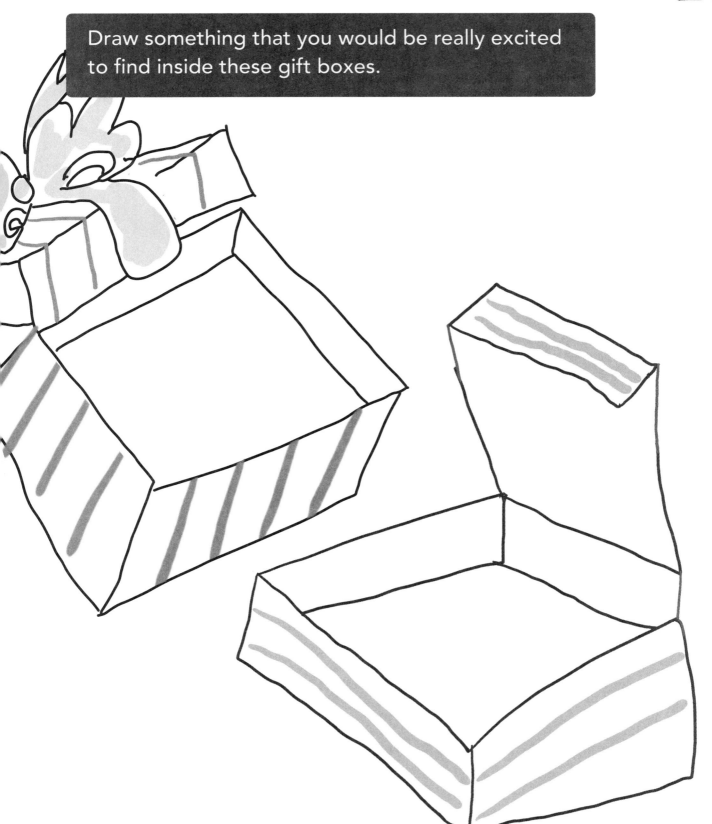

Get excited! Fill in the blanks.

Imagine you just found a bag of gold.

The number of gold coins is _____.

You will eat your favorite food.

The food is _____.

You just got the pet you wanted.

The pet is a _____.

Peep's pet, Goldie

You will spend the day with someone special.

That person is _____.

These children are excited. Draw their excited faces and jumping feet.

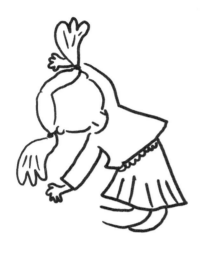

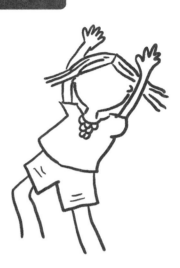

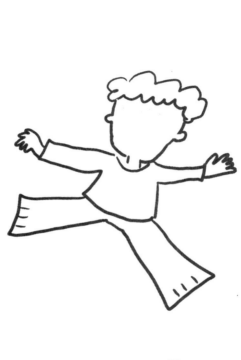

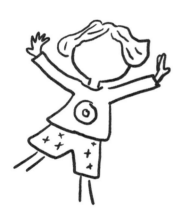

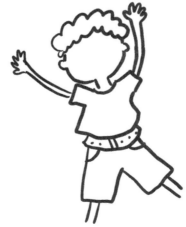

SCHOOL FAIR DREAMS
FEELING #7

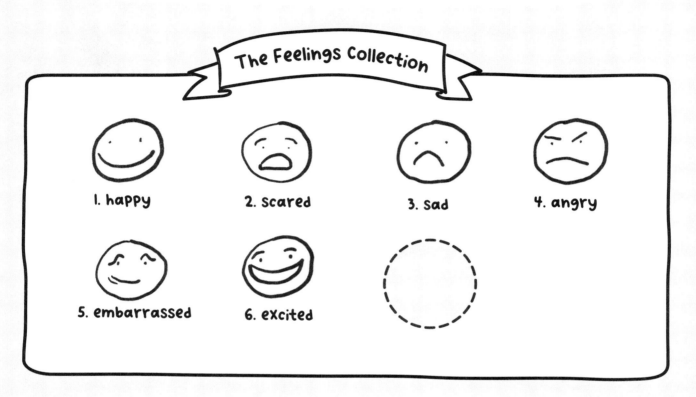

The Feelings Collection

1. happy
2. scared
3. sad
4. angry
5. embarrassed
6. excited

ARE YOU READY TO NAME THE NEXT FEELING?

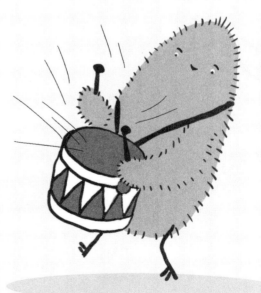

On Wednesday, it was the School Fair. During the School Fair, the school has rides, games, and food trucks instead of having classes. I was so excited for the fair!

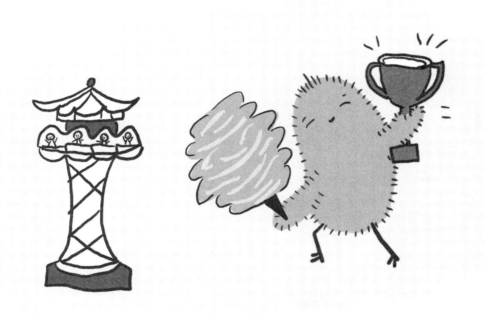

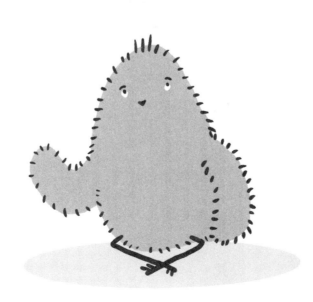

I planned to ride The Big Drop. Last year, I was too short to go on it.

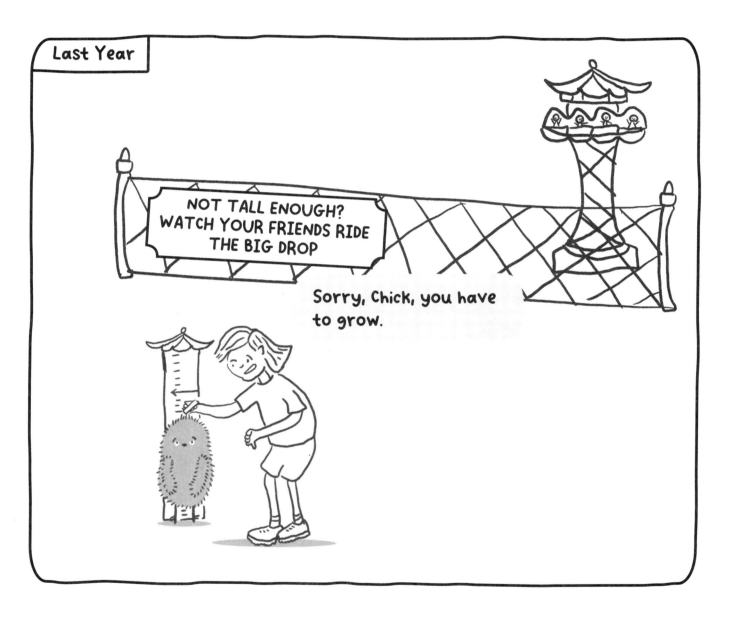

This year, I'm tall enough to go on the ride!

I also planned to buy cotton candy for J. J. Scruffles, my best friend. And I wanted to ride the Ferris Wheel with my friend Square, the starfish. Square is still too short to ride The Big Drop.

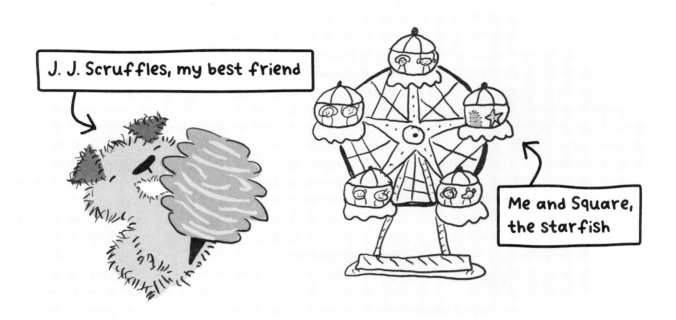

J. J. Scruffles, my best friend

Me and Square, the starfish

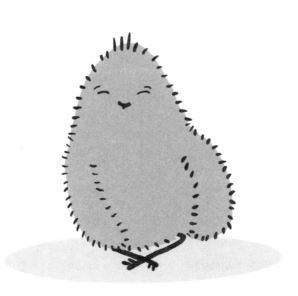

How much money did Peep bring to the fair? Add up the amounts.

Peep's Money Collection

Birthday money

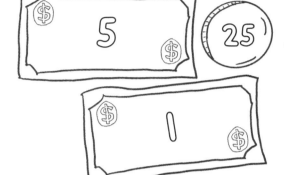

$ _____ . _____

Money made from helping Aunt Gina collect eggs

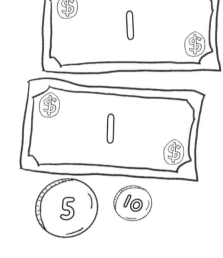

Allowance money

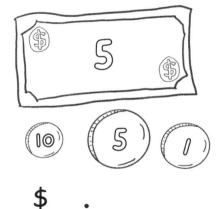

$ _____ . _____

$ _____ . _____

ALL PEEP'S MONEY TOGETHER = $ _____ . _____

ANSWER: Birthday money: $6.25 Allowance: $5.16 Egg money: $2.15, Total: $13.56

38.

On my way to school, it started pouring rain. When I got to school, a sign said the School Fair was off. We had to go to class just like any other day.

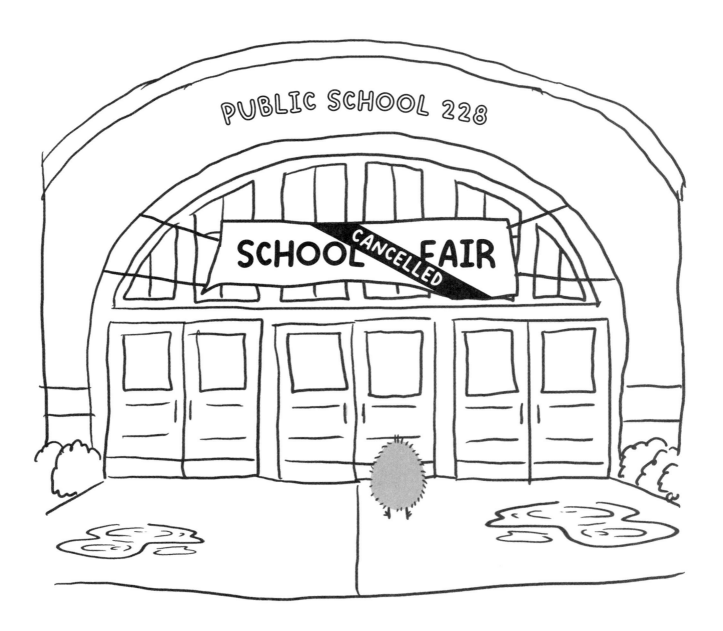

I dragged myself to my classroom. I fought hard to hold back my tears.

I was feeling…

_____

Write the feeling on the line.

I tried not to cry. I wanted to hide my disappointment.

Have you ever tried to hide your feelings?

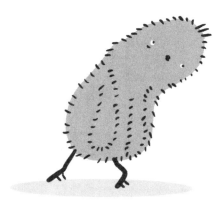

ANSWER: Disappointed
Or other feelings—like upset or frustrated

40.

Finish drawing the disappointed faces.

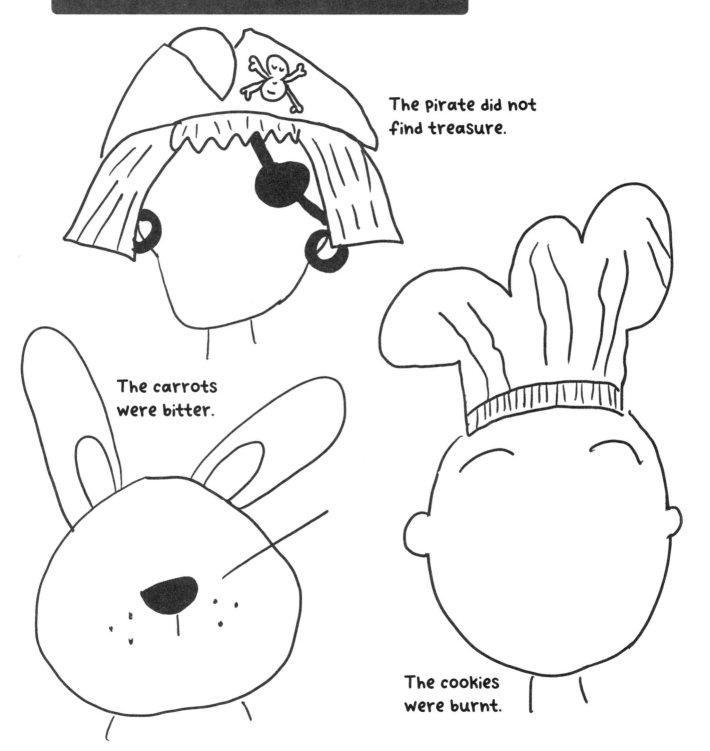

The pirate did not find treasure.

The carrots were bitter.

The cookies were burnt.

41.

Draw the **opposite** of disappointed faces.

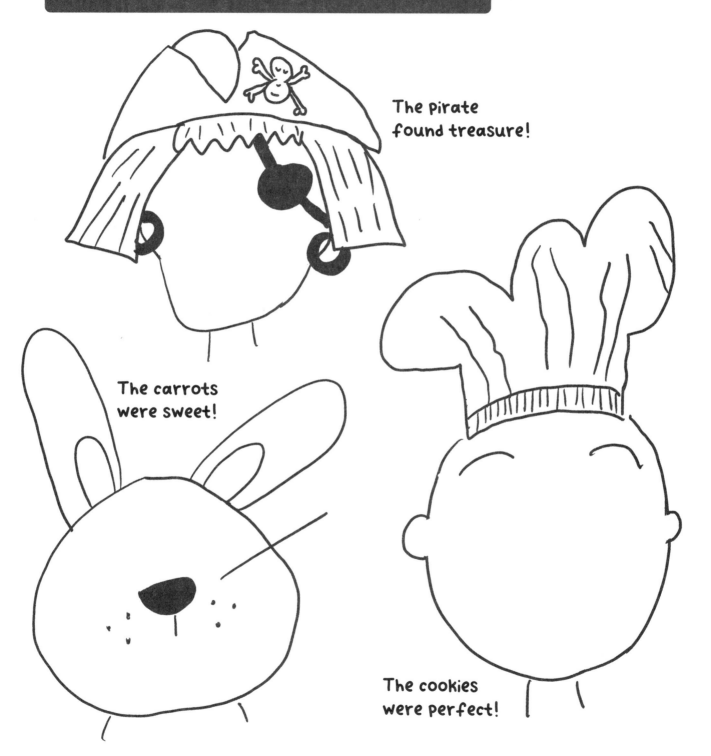

The pirate found treasure!

The carrots were sweet!

The cookies were perfect!

Ask three people to tell you a story about a time they felt disappointed. Then, ask them to rate the size of their disappointment on the feelings-o-meter.

Story of

feelings-o-meter rating

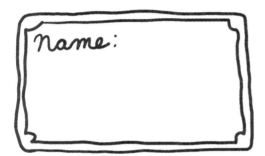

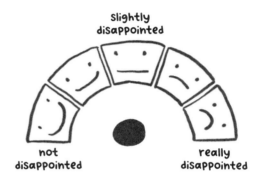

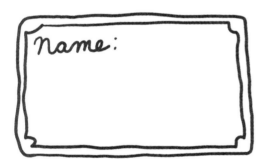

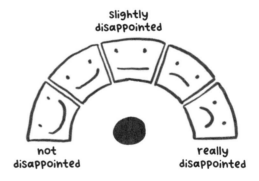

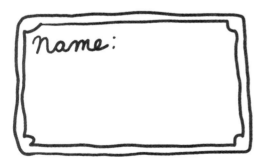

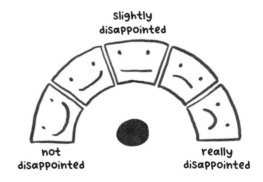

TALENT SHOW JITTERS
FEELING #8

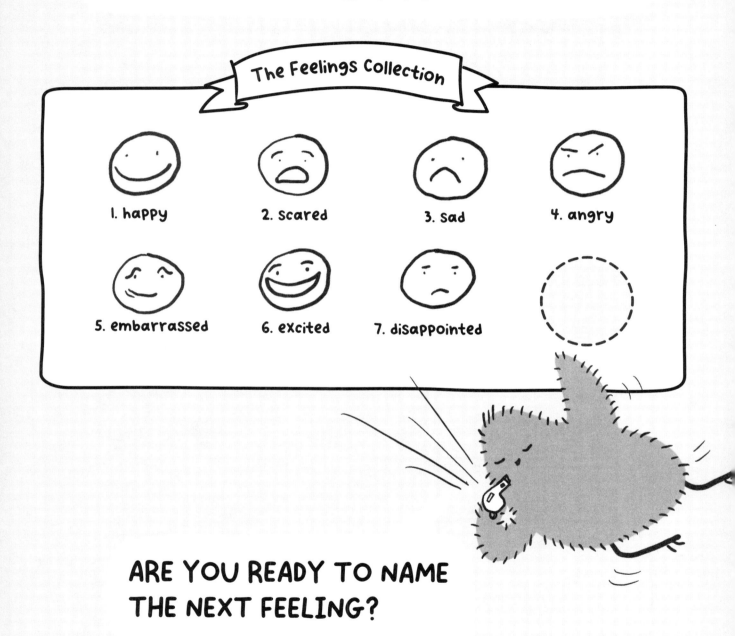

ARE YOU READY TO NAME
THE NEXT FEELING?

On Thursday, it was the talent show. My friends were excited to be on stage.

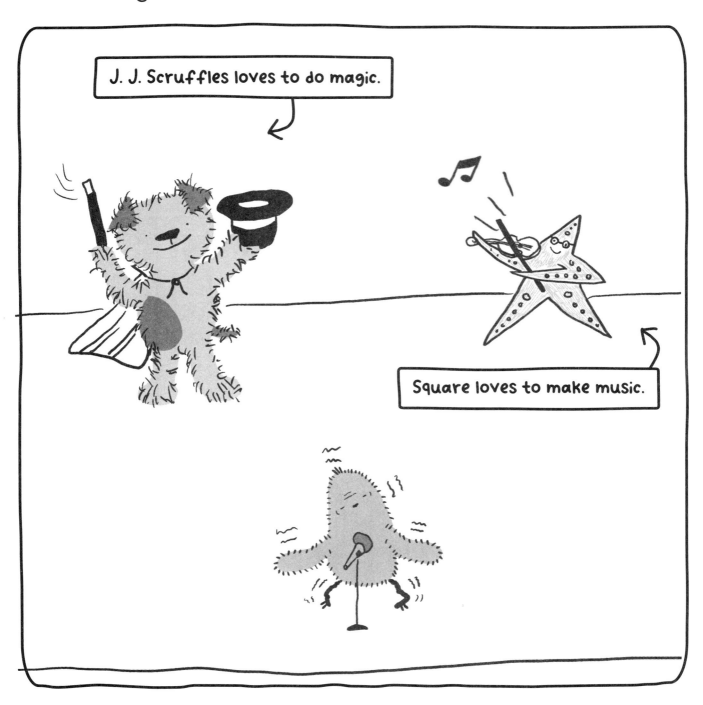

I did not want to be on stage!

I did not want to be in the talent show, but my music teacher said I had a good voice. So I told the teacher that I would take a risk and sing on stage.

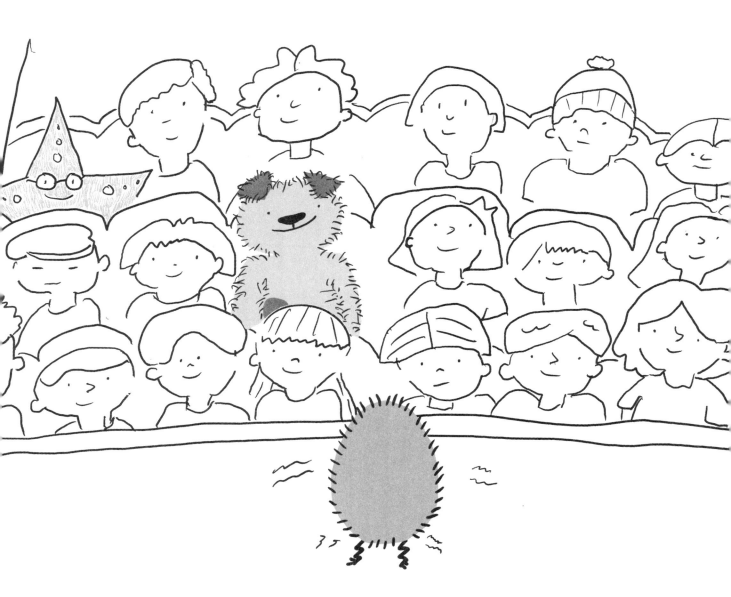

Help the kids to hear Peep sing. Draw the missing ears.

At first, my tummy was all twisted in knots and my legs felt like they were made of jelly.

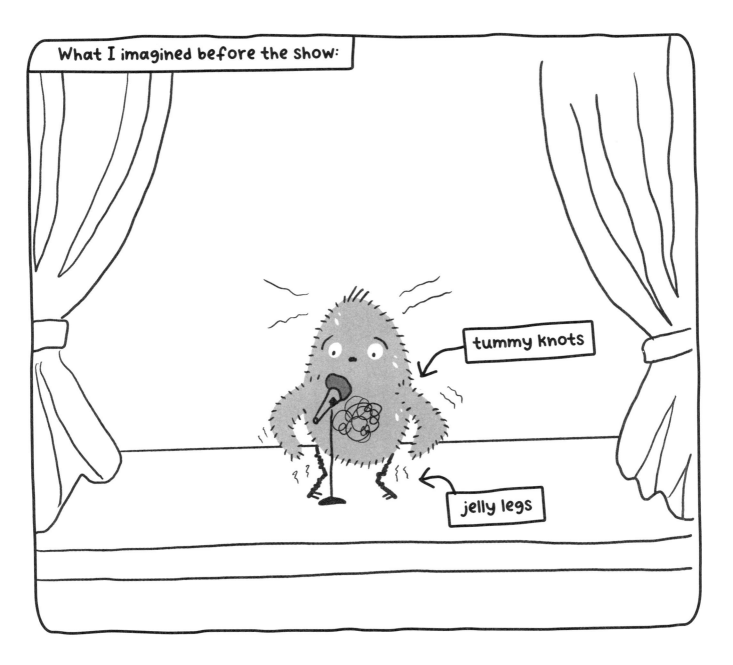

What I imagined before the show:

tummy knots

jelly legs

I tried to sing, but no words came out. But then, things got better. My tummy stopped twisting and my legs felt stronger. I sang loud!

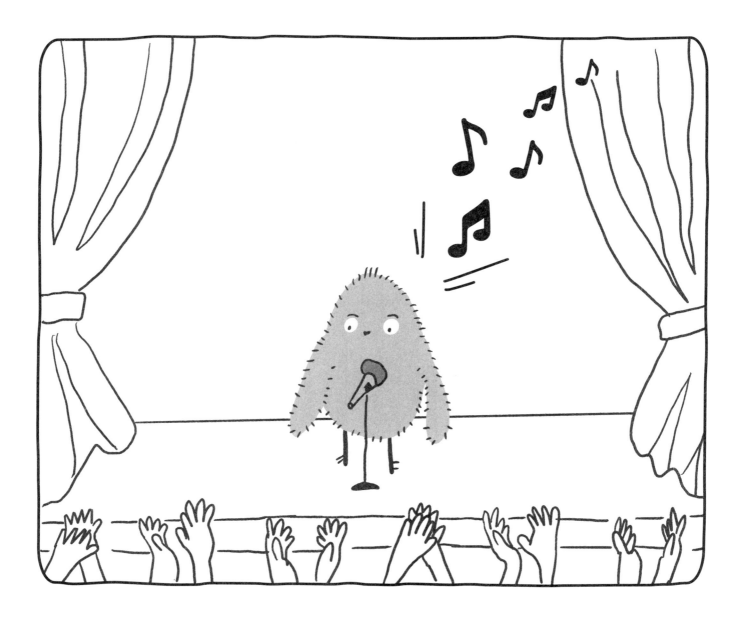

Soon, my song was done. When I took a bow, my breath was slow and steady. Everyone clapped for me.

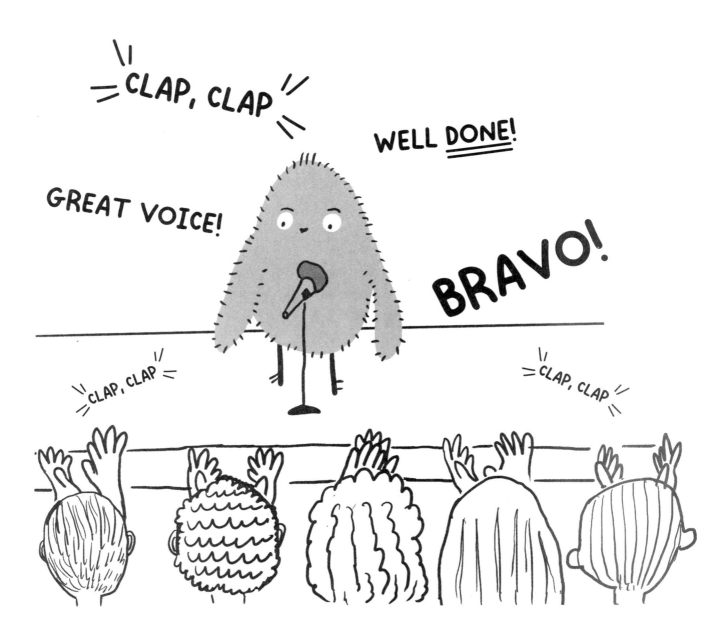

I was feeling...

_____

Write the feeling on the line.

Great work! Our collection
keeps growing!

And did you notice? My
feelings changed. How was
I feeling before I sang?

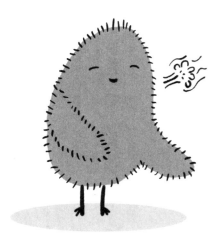

ANSWER: Relieved
Or other feelings—like calm, relaxed, pleased

Peep's tummy was filled with knots before he sang.
Fill the page with knots.

BEFORE:

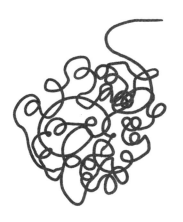

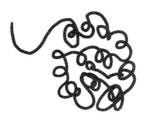

Peep's tummy knots went away after he sang.
Untangle the knots.

AFTER:

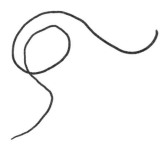

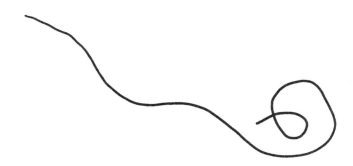

The foot didn't step on the ants. The ants are relieved. Draw their faces.

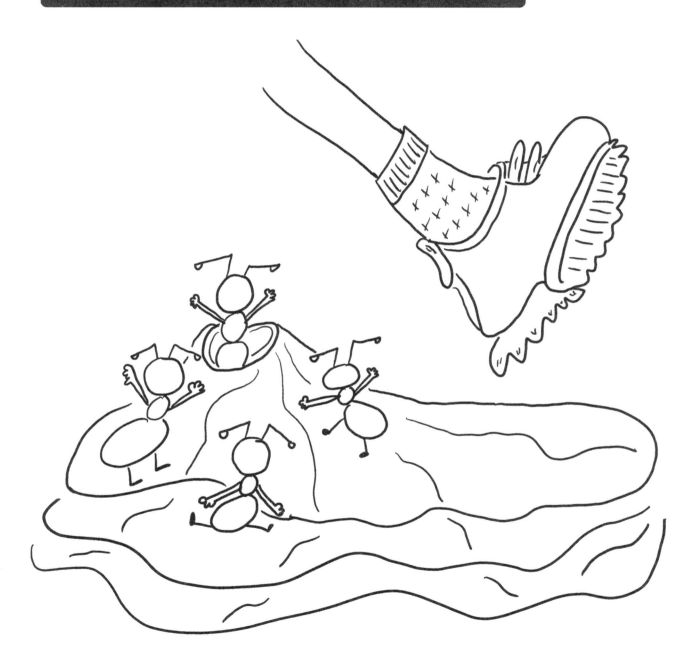

The kids are relieved. Draw them exhaling, letting their breath out.

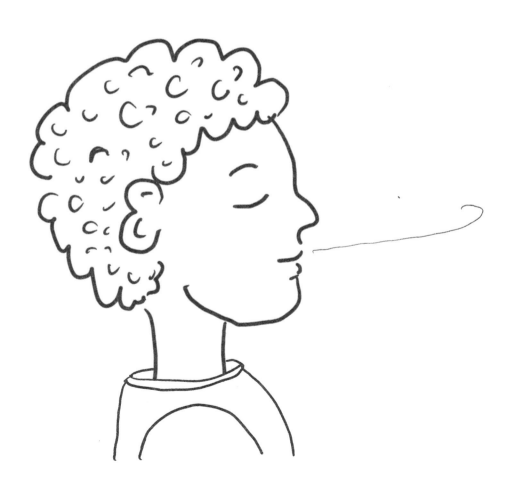

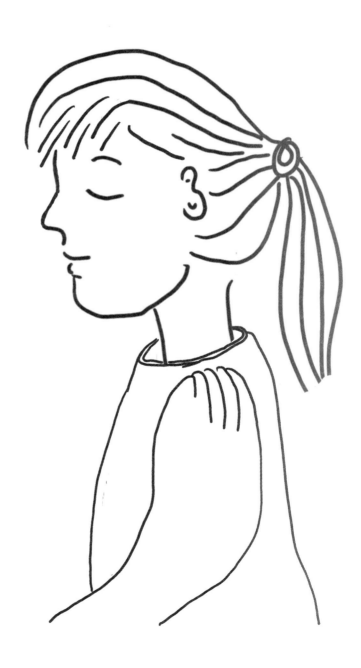

MONSTER CHECK MADNESS
FEELING #9

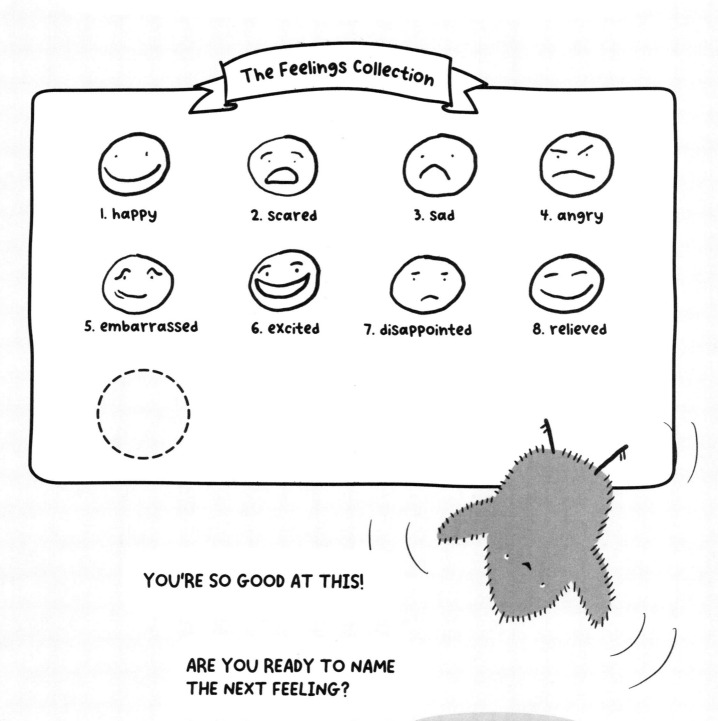

The Feelings Collection

1. happy
2. scared
3. sad
4. angry
5. embarrassed
6. excited
7. disappointed
8. relieved

YOU'RE SO GOOD AT THIS!

ARE YOU READY TO NAME
THE NEXT FEELING?

On Friday, before I went to bed, I checked my room for monsters. My heart beats fast when I do the "monster check."

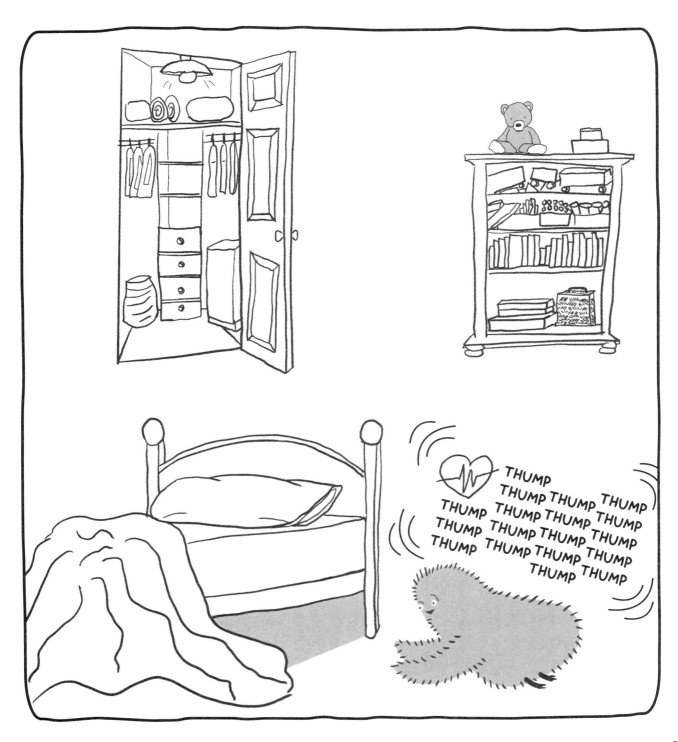

I know monsters aren't real. But I still do my "monster check!" I look in all the places on my list and say, "Boo!" I scare the monsters away before they can scare me!

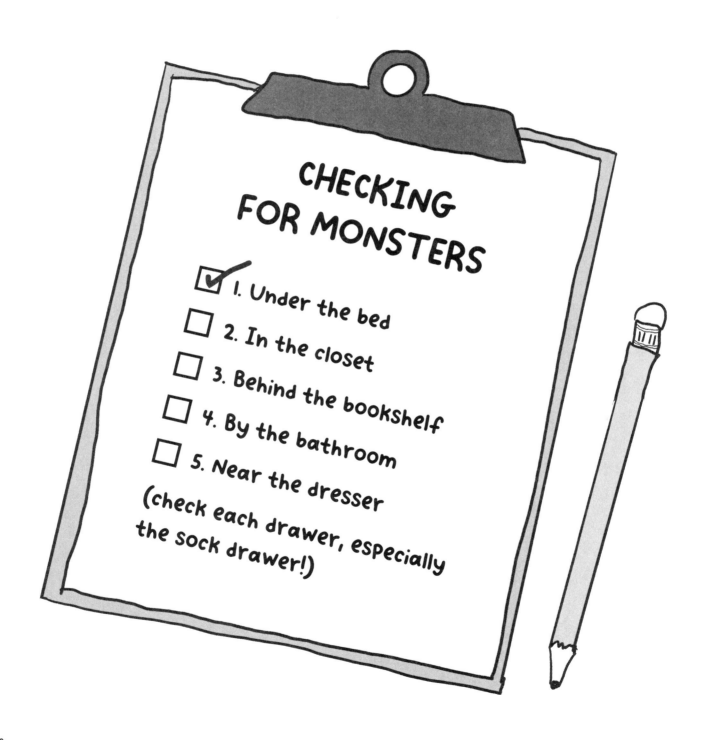

CHECKING FOR MONSTERS

☑ 1. Under the bed
☐ 2. In the closet
☐ 3. Behind the bookshelf
☐ 4. By the bathroom
☐ 5. Near the dresser
(check each drawer, especially the sock drawer!)

I also sleep with my "monster protectors" close by. These things protect me from monsters and other scary things.

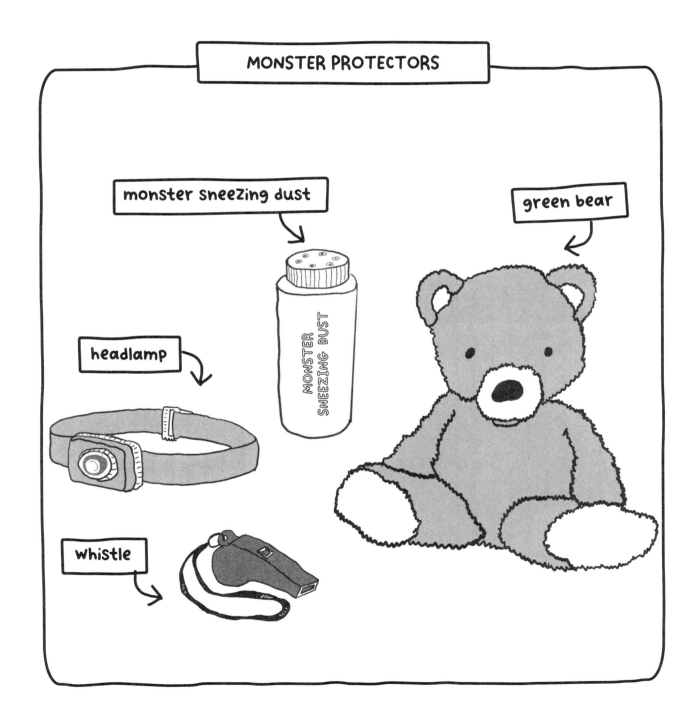

After I checked for monsters, I climbed into bed, but I couldn't fall asleep. My arms and legs felt a little shaky. Thoughts about monsters swirled around in my head.

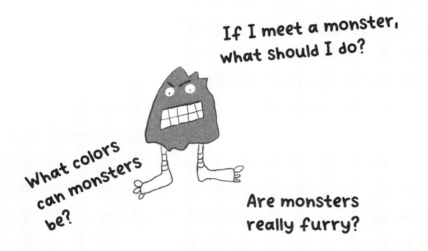

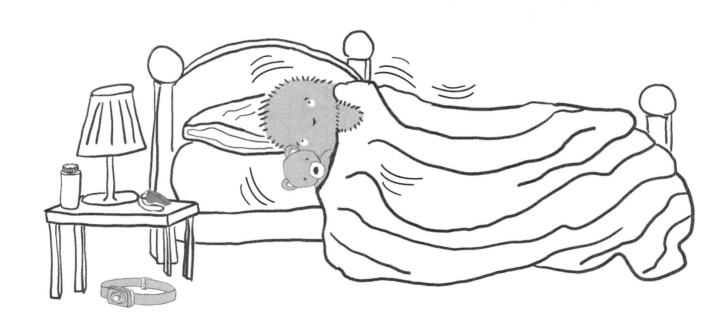

I was feeling….

_____

Write the feeling on the line.

Rate the size of Peep's worry.

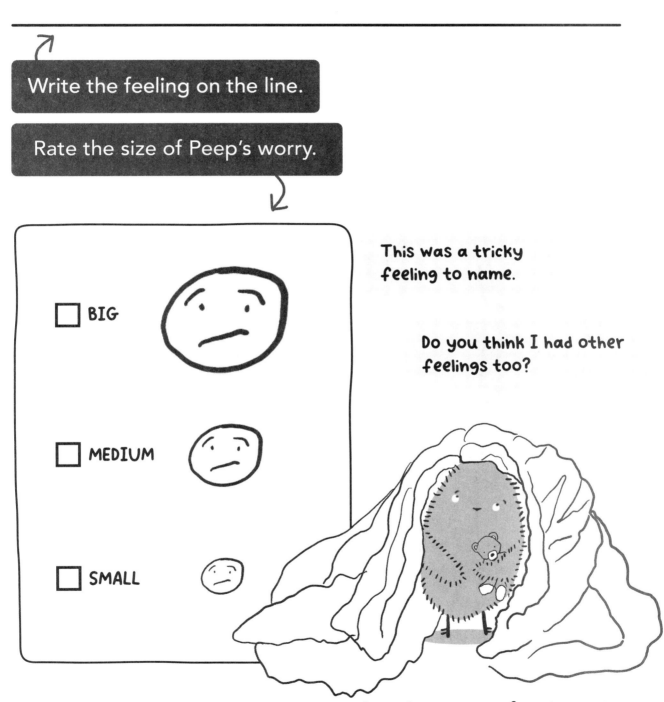

☐ BIG

☐ MEDIUM

☐ SMALL

This was a tricky feeling to name.

Do you think I had other feelings too?

Or other feelings—like nervous, tense, anxious
ANSWER: Worried

61.

Fill the sack with things that help you feel safe when you are worried.

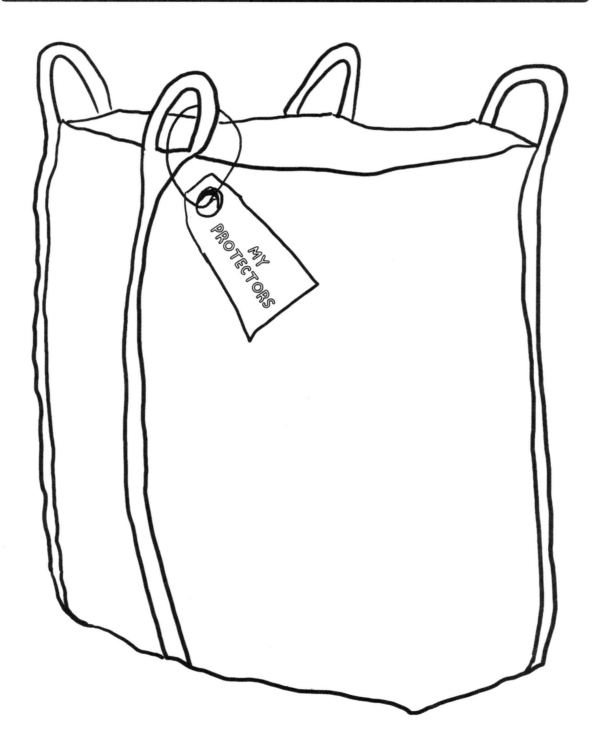

MY PROTECTORS

Five of these cats are worried. Five of them are asleep. Draw the eyes on the cats.

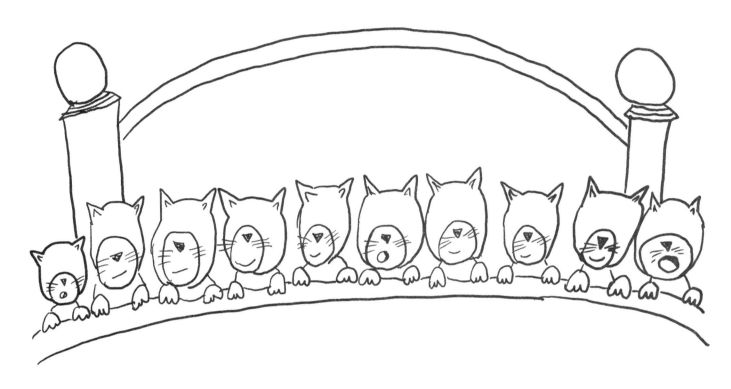

Here are some feeling words that are similar to "worry." Unscramble them.

1. DAFRIA   _ _ _ _ _ _

2. SNERVOU   _ _ _ _ _ _ _

3. NISAXOU   _ _ _ _ _ _ _

4. DESCAR   _ _ _ _ _ _

5. YEASNU   _ _ _ _ _ _

Make up a recipe for Monster Sneezing Dust.

HOW TO MAKE MONSTER SNEEZING DUST

First, add 2 pinches of _____.
(noun)

Next, mix in I spoonful of _____.
(noun)

After, _____ and add ½ cup of _____.
(verb)   (noun)

Finally, _____ and say the words _____,
(verb)   (noun)

_____, and _____.
(noun)   (noun)

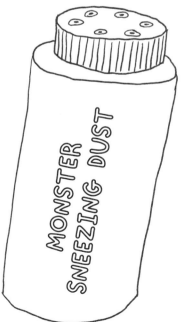

(noun) = person, place, or thing
(verb) = action word

SUPER SOCCER SUCCESS
FEELING #10

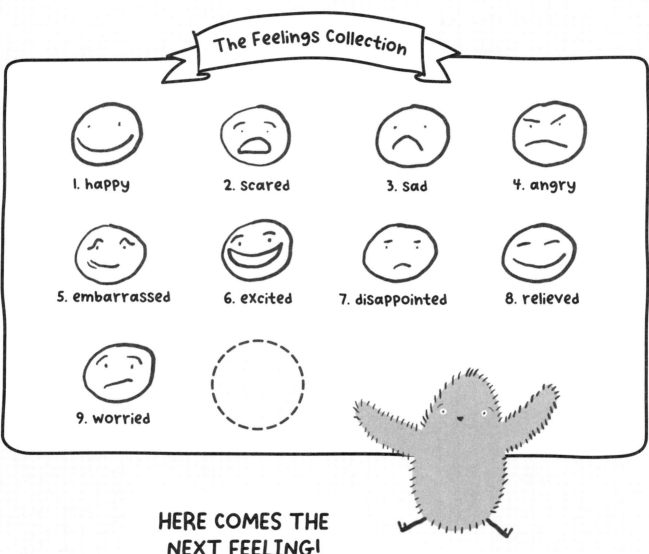

The Feelings Collection

1. happy
2. scared
3. sad
4. angry
5. embarrassed
6. excited
7. disappointed
8. relieved
9. worried

HERE COMES THE
NEXT FEELING!

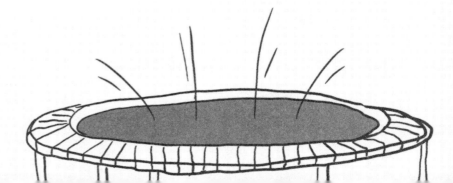

On Saturday, my soccer team, the Big Foot Stompers, crushed the Kicking Bandits. The score was 3-1. I passed two balls to my friend Flo. She kicked them right into the goal!

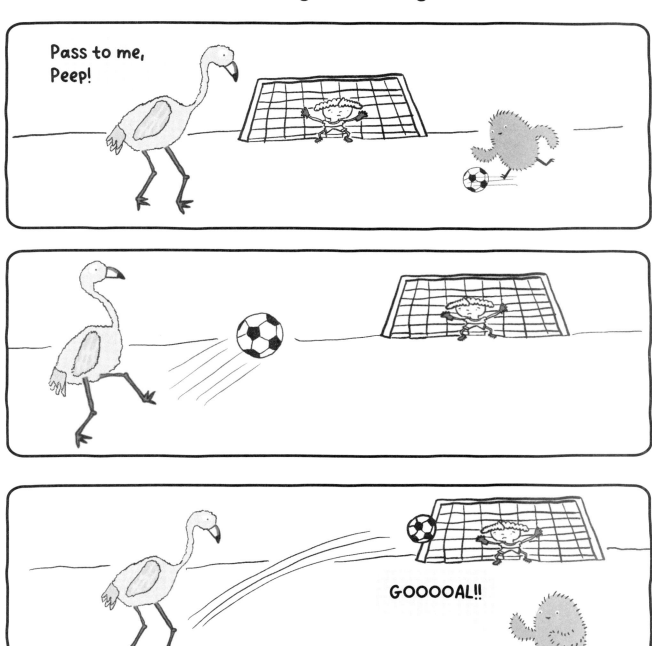

After each game, Coach Robin gives an award to the star of the game. I don't listen because I never win it. Instead, I think about ice cream.

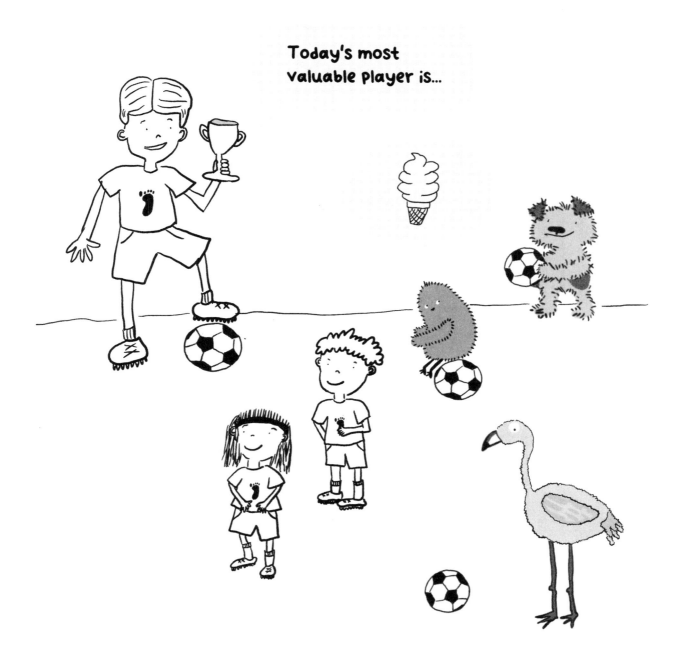

Today's most valuable player is...

When I won the award, I was too busy thinking about ice cream. Coach Robin had to shout my name to get my attention.

Peep!

Peep!

...Peep!

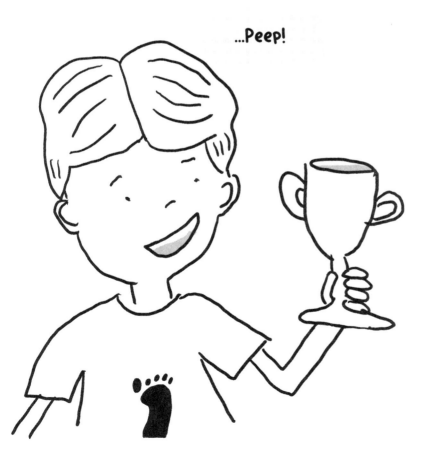

My teammates cheered like crazy for me.

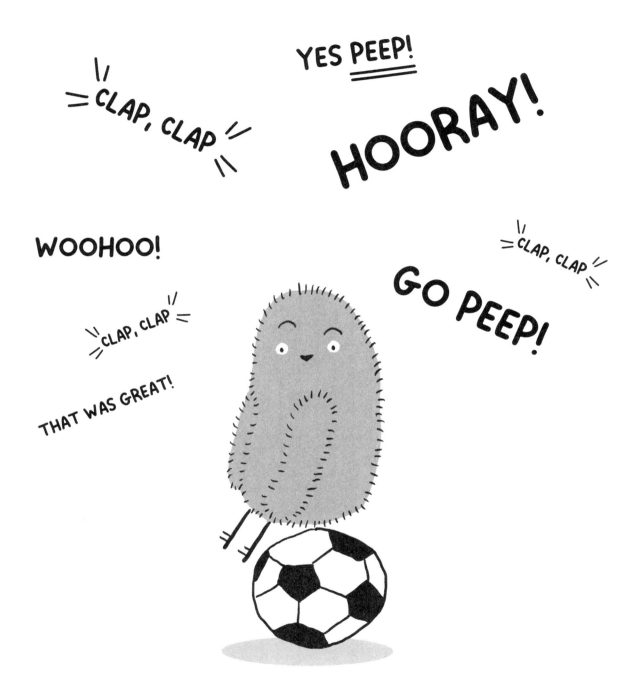

When Coach Robin said my name, I froze for a moment.

I was feeling…

_____

↗

Write the feeling on the line.

Have you ever
felt surprised?

How did it make your
body feel?

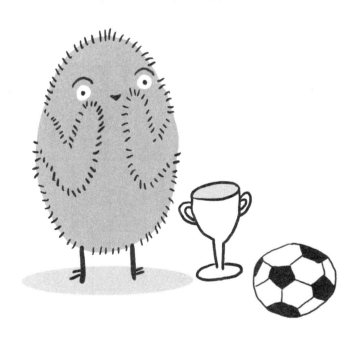

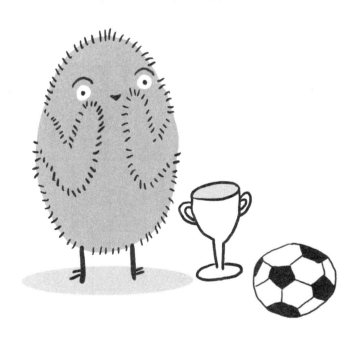

ANSWER: Surprised
or other feelings—like shocked, amazed, stunned

The team with the most goals will be surprised! Find the winning team!

SEASON SCOREBOARD

	Goals			Goals
The Turbo Turtles	3	VS.	The Crazy Cleats	1
The Jellybean Jugglers	2	VS.	The Turbo Turtles	3
The Crazy Cleats	2	VS.	The Kickin' Kangaroos	1
The Kickin' Kangaroos	3	VS.	The Jellybean Jugglers	2

Team	Number of Goals

There is a surprise in the room. Draw it.

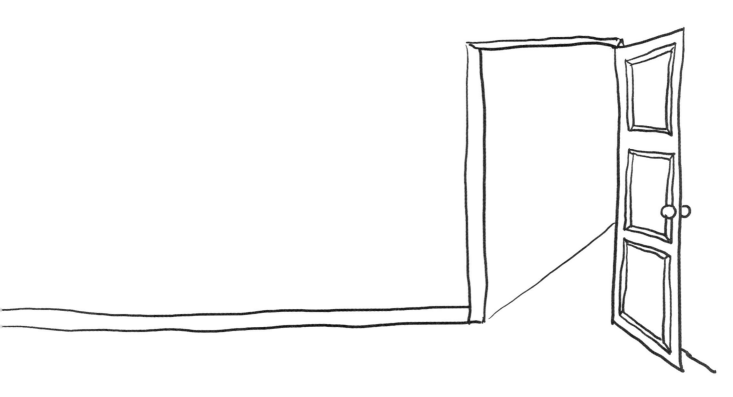

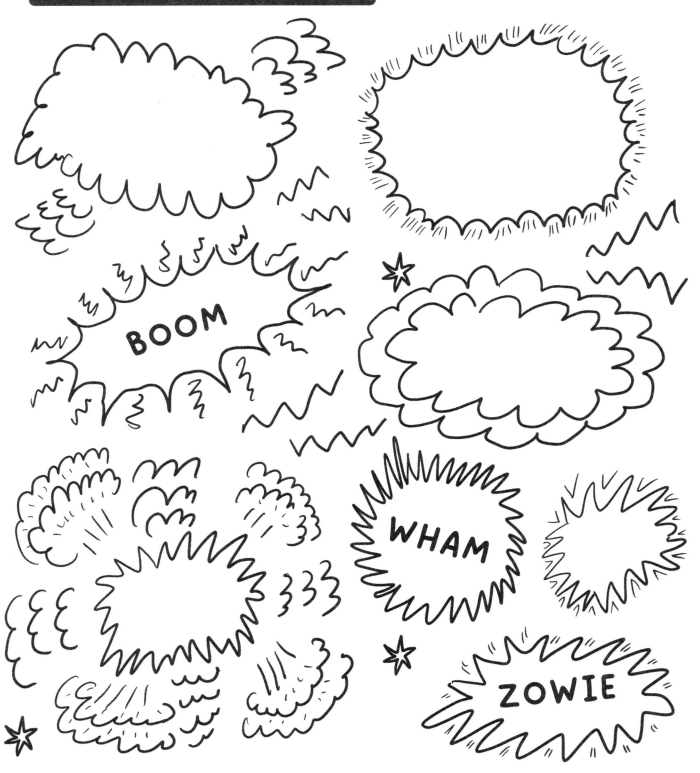

Surprise someone with an amazing cake.
Finish decorating it.

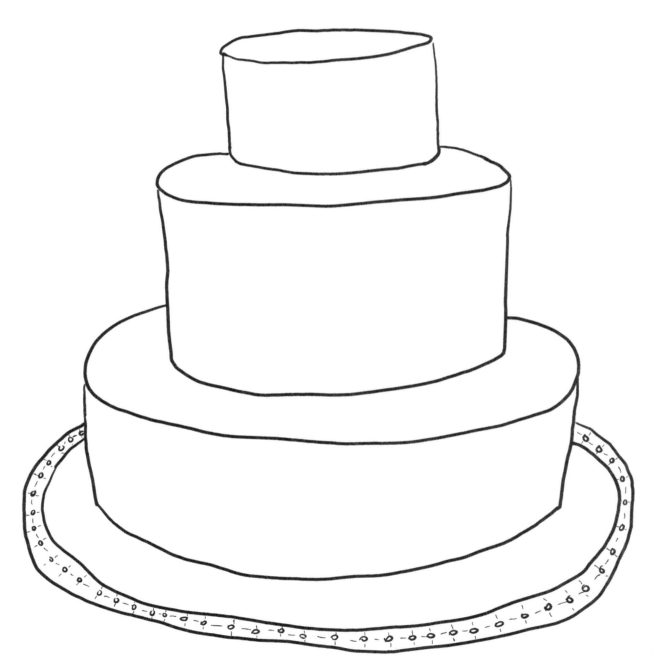

PLAYDATE PLANS CHANGE
FEELING #11

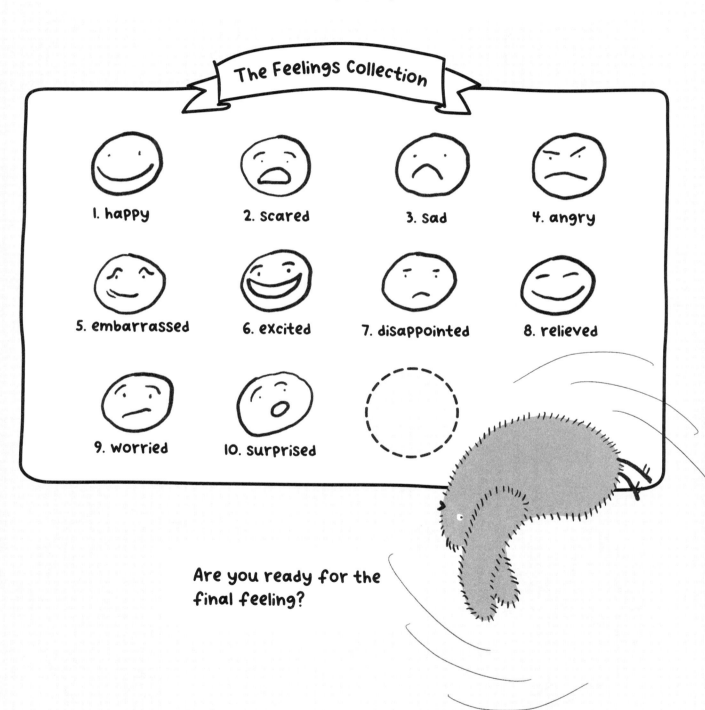

The Feelings Collection

1. happy
2. scared
3. sad
4. angry
5. embarrassed
6. excited
7. disappointed
8. relieved
9. worried
10. surprised

Are you ready for the final feeling?

On Sunday, J. J. Scruffles, my best friend, was coming to my house to play. I planned our day.

10:00 AM	Trade Sharky Shark Cards
10:45 AM	Play Block City
11:30 AM	Build Galaxy Blaster
12:00 PM	LUNCH
1:00 PM	Play with Mole Crickets
1:30 PM	Kick Soccer Balls
2:30 PM	SNACK
3:00 PM	J. J. Goes Home

I was looking at my Sharky Shark trading cards when I heard Gran calling for me.

Peep. Peep. There's been a change.

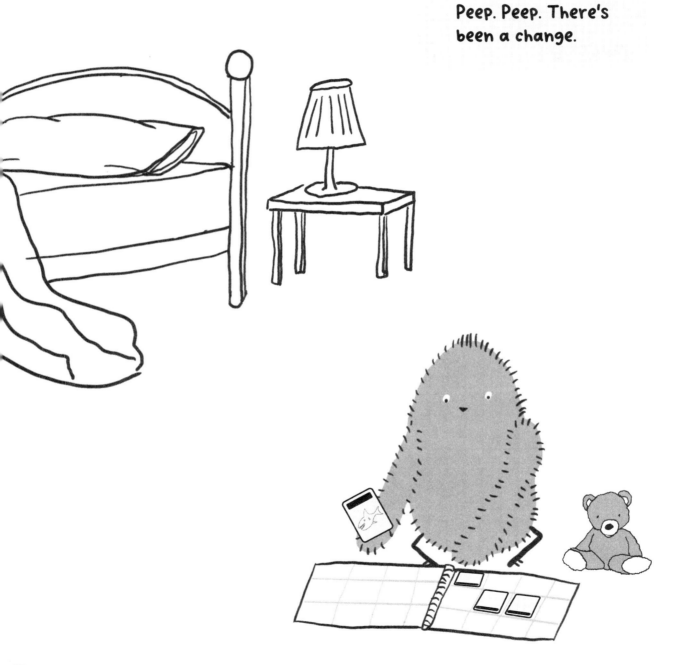

Gran came into my room to tell me about the change.

I'm sorry Peep, but J. J. Scruffles can't come to play today. He had to go to his sister's swim meet.

The whole day?

Yes, the whole day.
He cannot play today.

Can I invite Flo over?

Flo is food shopping with her dad.

How about Square.
Can we call Square?

Square is with his grandmom.

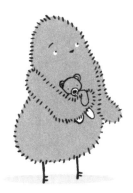

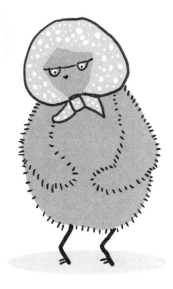

When Gran left my room, I flopped onto my bed. There was nothing fun to do by myself. I wanted to be with a friend.

• • • • • • • •

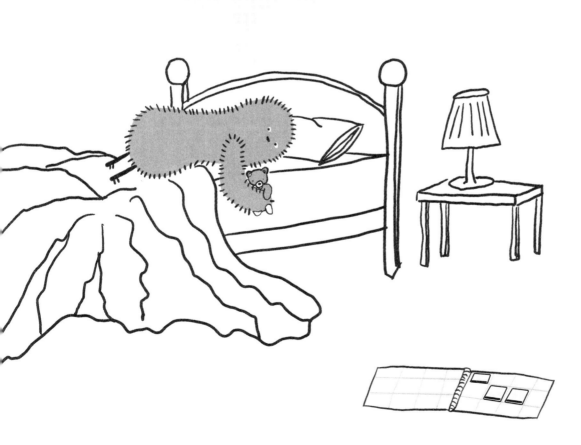

I was feeling....

_____

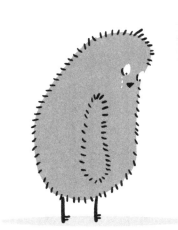

Write the feeling on the line.

It is okay to feel
lonely sometimes.

All feelings are okay.
Feelings are like
hearing the news. It
tells you something.

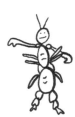

ANSWER: Lonely
Or other feelings—like empty, friendless, left out

One cat is lonely. Two cats are not. Draw their faces.

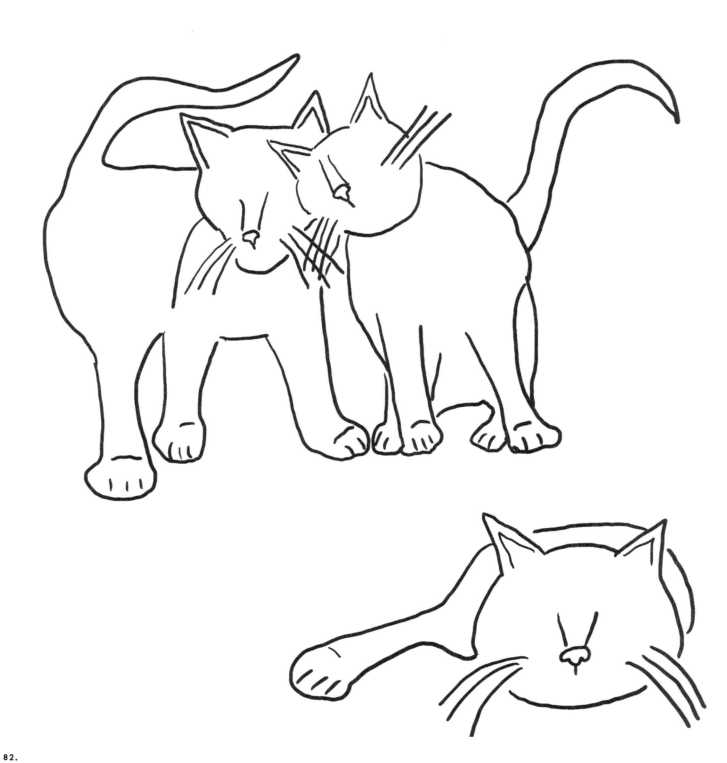

Think of a friend that you'd like to blow bubbles with. Fill the page with bubbles.

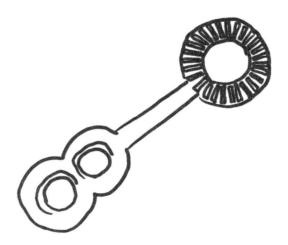

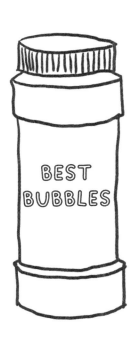

BEST
BUBBLES

OUR FEELINGS!

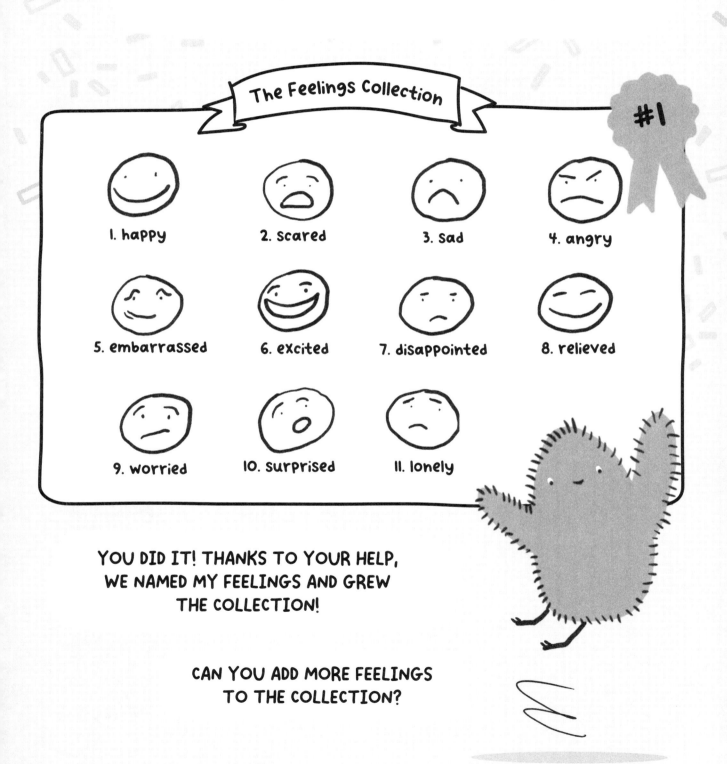

The Feelings Collection

#1

1. happy
2. scared
3. sad
4. angry
5. embarrassed
6. excited
7. disappointed
8. relieved
9. worried
10. surprised
11. lonely

YOU DID IT! THANKS TO YOUR HELP,
WE NAMED MY FEELINGS AND GREW
THE COLLECTION!

CAN YOU ADD MORE FEELINGS
TO THE COLLECTION?

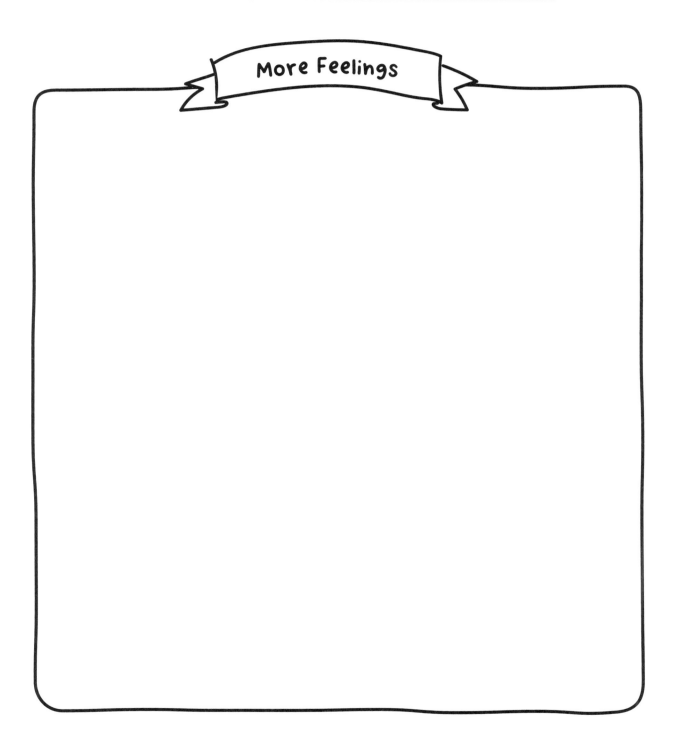

More Feelings

Circle AGREE or DISAGREE.

1. Every feeling has a name, like "sad," "happy," or "angry."

AGREE   DISAGREE

2. Feelings make our bodies feel a certain way, like TIGHT, TINGLY, or JUMPY.

AGREE   DISAGREE

3. We can share our feelings with people, or we can hide them.

AGREE   DISAGREE

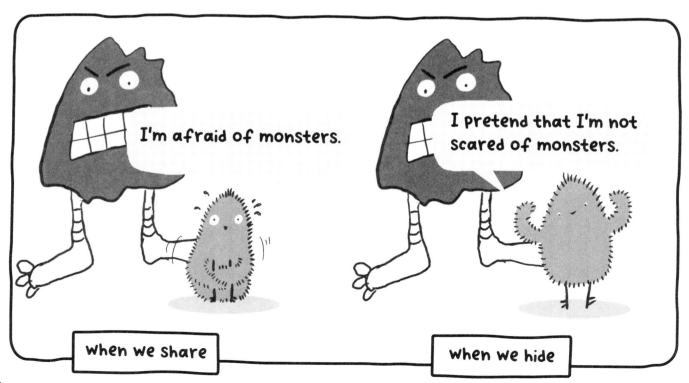

4. Feelings can change quickly.

   AGREE   DISAGREE

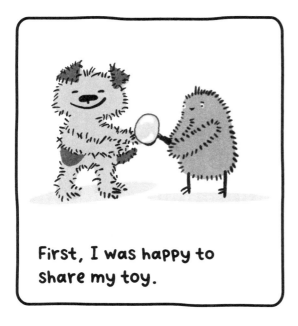

First, I was happy to share my toy.

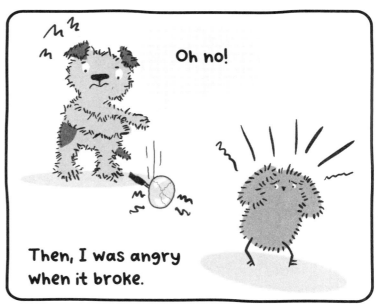

Oh no!

Then, I was angry when it broke.

5. There are no right or wrong feelings.

   AGREE   DISAGREE

feelings-o-meter

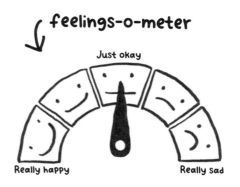

6. Feelings can be strong or weak.

   AGREE   DISAGREE

7. We can have more than one feeling at the same time.

   AGREE   DISAGREE

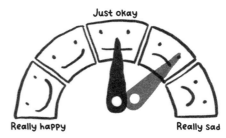

You are really smart about feelings.
You helped me feel smart too.

**YOU'RE THE WORLD'S GREATEST
COLLECTOR OF FEELINGS!**

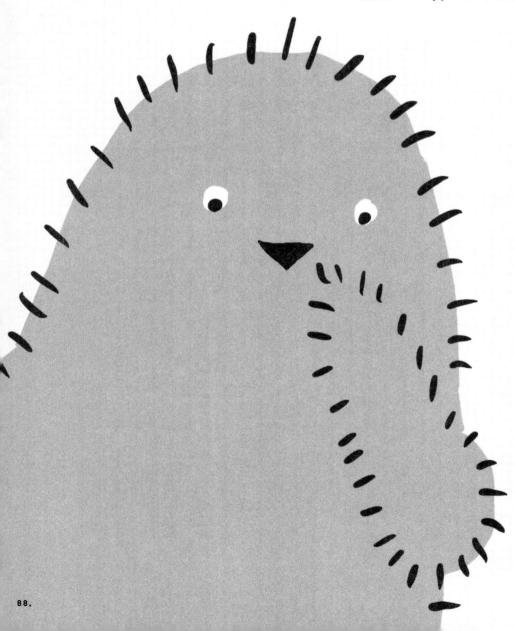

LETTER TO ADULTS

Dear adults,

The Big Book of Big Feelings is here to help children develop both literacy and emotional intelligence. When these two skills come together, they make a big difference—they help kids better understand, talk about, and manage their feelings.

Both literacy and emotional intelligence are key life skills that need nurturing, guidance, and practice. Fiction, especially, helps children to build these skills, along with their capacity for empathy, compassion, and self-reflection, all in a fun and engaging way. Through the magic of reading, a kid's senses come alive! They dive into books and explore new worlds full of interesting characters, exciting places, and big ideas. In *The Big Book of Big Feelings*, they'll meet characters like Peep, who will show them how to navigate emotions and learn from the outcomes of their actions.

Peep invites children to expand their vocabulary beyond common feeling words like "happy," "sad," and "angry," and helps them discover a whole new set of emotions. By learning more precise words for their feelings, kids can express themselves more clearly. When they have the tools to communicate better, they're understood more easily, which strengthens relationships and helps them grow into kinder, more thoughtful individuals.

Here are some fun ways to use this book to help a child you care for grow in both literacy and emotional intelligence. These tips can make it easier for them to share how they're feeling with the people around them.

- **Read together, or let them take the lead.** If your child isn't reading on their own yet, read the book aloud to them. If they are reading on their own, ask if they'd prefer to read by themselves or with you. If you're reading together, take turns. When your child reads aloud, listen closely, and gently correct any tricky words or ideas they might stumble over. (It's okay to let small mistakes slide.) They might read slower than you'd expect at first, but with time, they'll get faster and more confident.

- **Get involved!** Dive into the activity pages together, and ask your child questions about Peep's adventures. For example, when you get to page 16, where Peep feels embarrassed about burping out loud, ask your child if they've ever felt embarrassed. Then, share a time you were embarrassed, too. It's a wonderful way to bond, and hearing and sharing personal stories helps children understand emotions better.

- **Listen first.** Instead of telling your child how they should feel, focus on hearing what they say about their own emotions. By doing this, you'll learn more about their inner world, and maybe even notice when they need help finding the right words to express themselves.

- **Watch for the pencil icon!** This symbol marks the activity pages. After completing them, encourage your child to get creative—color the page or add extra details to make it their own.

- **Let them draw their way.** When they're working on an activity page, avoid telling them how to draw or what to do. Some kids can feel shy about their drawing skills, so it's better to cheer them on and let them create freely.

- **Use the tips on pages 9 and 10** as a guide for having meaningful conversations about emotions with your child.

Last thing: While I've said "your child" above, which often connotes a parent, this book is for teachers, caregivers, and any other adult who works with children or cares for a child in their lives.

Have fun!

Rachael Katz

Rachael Katz

Rachael Katz, MEd, has over twenty-five years of experience as an educator, school leader, and program developer for children. She made her career choice at just six years old—after spending a day on a children's television show counting with a furry, blue monster who loved cookies. From that day on, she knew she wanted to work in education and make learning fun.

Rachael's experience includes serving as head of the Discovery School at the Bay Area Discovery Museum, leading social and emotional learning for Early Years at Dulwich College Beijing, and teaching preschool through third grade in both public and private schools. Beyond the classroom, Rachael has created and written television content for Nick Jr. and Radio Television Hong Kong, and consulted on educational programming for the Children's Television Workshop. She has also designed educational toys for Baby Care Limited and the Child Growth and Development Corporation. Rachael is coauthor of The Emotionally Intelligent Child. She is currently writing a series of children's books focused on emotional literacy.

She holds a master's degree in education from Bank Street College, and a BA from the Tisch School of the Arts at New York University.

MORE BOOKS from
NEW HARBINGER PUBLICATIONS

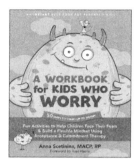
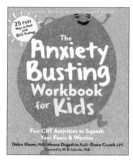
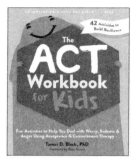
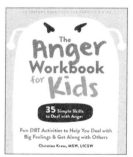
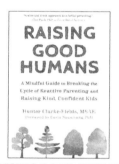
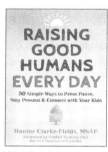